Adaptive Designs for Sequential Treatment Allocation

Chapman & Hall/CRC Biostatistics Series

Editor-in-Chief

Shein-Chung Chow, Ph.D., Professor, Department of Biostatistics and Bioinformatics, Duke University School of Medicine, Durham, North Carolina

Series Editors

Byron Jones, Biometrical Fellow, Statistical Methodology, Integrated Information Sciences, Novartis Pharma AG, Basel, Switzerland

Jen-pei Liu, Professor, Division of Biometry, Department of Agronomy, National Taiwan University, Taipei, Taiwan

Karl E. Peace, Georgia Cancer Coalition, Distinguished Cancer Scholar, Senior Research Scientist and Professor of Biostatistics, Jiann-Ping Hsu College of Public Health, Georgia Southern University, Statesboro, Georgia

Bruce W. Turnbull, Professor, School of Operations Research and Industrial Engineering, Cornell University, Ithaca, New York

Published Titles

Adaptive Design Methods in Clinical Trials, Second Edition
Shein-Chung Chow and Mark Chang

Adaptive Designs for Sequential Treatment Allocation
Alessandro Baldi Antognini and Alessandra Giovagnoli

Adaptive Design Theory and Implementation Using SAS and R, Second Edition
Mark Chang

Advanced Bayesian Methods for Medical Test Accuracy
Lyle D. Broemeling

Advances in Clinical Trial Biostatistics
Nancy L. Geller

Applied Meta-Analysis with R
Ding-Geng (Din) Chen and Karl E. Peace

Basic Statistics and Pharmaceutical Statistical Applications, Second Edition
James E. De Muth

Bayesian Adaptive Methods for Clinical Trials
Scott M. Berry, Bradley P. Carlin, J. Jack Lee, and Peter Muller

Bayesian Analysis Made Simple: An Excel GUI for WinBUGS
Phil Woodward

Bayesian Methods for Measures of Agreement
Lyle D. Broemeling

Bayesian Methods in Epidemiology
Lyle D. Broemeling

Bayesian Methods in Health Economics
Gianluca Baio

Bayesian Missing Data Problems: EM, Data Augmentation and Noniterative Computation
Ming T. Tan, Guo-Liang Tian, and Kai Wang Ng

Bayesian Modeling in Bioinformatics
Dipak K. Dey, Samiran Ghosh, and Bani K. Mallick

Benefit-Risk Assessment in Pharmaceutical Research and Development
Andreas Sashegyi, James Felli, and Rebecca Noel

Biosimilars: Design and Analysis of Follow-on Biologics
Shein-Chung Chow

Biostatistics: A Computing Approach
Stewart J. Anderson

Causal Analysis in Biomedicine and Epidemiology: Based on Minimal Sufficient Causation
Mikel Aickin

Clinical and Statistical Considerations in Personalized Medicine
Claudio Carini, Sandeep Menon, and Mark Chang

Clinical Trial Data Analysis using R
Ding-Geng (Din) Chen and Karl E. Peace

Clinical Trial Methodology
Karl E. Peace and Ding-Geng (Din) Chen

Computational Methods in Biomedical Research
Ravindra Khattree and Dayanand N. Naik

Computational Pharmacokinetics
Anders Källén

Confidence Intervals for Proportions and Related Measures of Effect Size
Robert G. Newcombe

Controversial Statistical Issues in Clinical Trials
Shein-Chung Chow

Data and Safety Monitoring Committees in Clinical Trials
Jay Herson

Design and Analysis of Animal Studies in Pharmaceutical Development
Shein-Chung Chow and Jen-pei Liu

Design and Analysis of Bioavailability and Bioequivalence Studies, Third Edition
Shein-Chung Chow and Jen-pei Liu

Design and Analysis of Bridging Studies
Jen-pei Liu, Shein-Chung Chow, and Chin-Fu Hsiao

Design and Analysis of Clinical Trials for Predictive Medicine
Shigeyuki Matsui, Marc Buyse, and Richard Simon

Design and Analysis of Clinical Trials with Time-to-Event Endpoints
Karl E. Peace

Design and Analysis of Non-Inferiority Trials
Mark D. Rothmann, Brian L. Wiens, and Ivan S. F. Chan

Difference Equations with Public Health Applications
Lemuel A. Moyé and Asha Seth Kapadia

DNA Methylation Microarrays: Experimental Design and Statistical Analysis
Sun-Chong Wang and Arturas Petronis

DNA Microarrays and Related Genomics Techniques: Design, Analysis, and Interpretation of Experiments
David B. Allison, Grier P. Page, T. Mark Beasley, and Jode W. Edwards

Dose Finding by the Continual Reassessment Method
Ying Kuen Cheung

Elementary Bayesian Biostatistics
Lemuel A. Moyé

Frailty Models in Survival Analysis
Andreas Wienke

Generalized Linear Models: A Bayesian Perspective
Dipak K. Dey, Sujit K. Ghosh, and Bani K. Mallick

Handbook of Regression and Modeling: Applications for the Clinical and Pharmaceutical Industries
Daryl S. Paulson

Inference Principles for Biostatisticians
Ian C. Marschner

Interval-Censored Time-to-Event Data: Methods and Applications
Ding-Geng (Din) Chen, Jianguo Sun, and Karl E. Peace

Joint Models for Longitudinal and Time-to-Event Data: With Applications in R
Dimitris Rizopoulos

Measures of Interobserver Agreement and Reliability, Second Edition
Mohamed M. Shoukri

Medical Biostatistics, Third Edition
A. Indrayan

Meta-Analysis in Medicine and Health Policy
Dalene Stangl and Donald A. Berry

Mixed Effects Models for the Population Approach: Models, Tasks, Methods and Tools
Marc Lavielle

Monte Carlo Simulation for the Pharmaceutical Industry: Concepts, Algorithms, and Case Studies
Mark Chang

Multiple Testing Problems in Pharmaceutical Statistics
Alex Dmitrienko, Ajit C. Tamhane, and Frank Bretz

Noninferiority Testing in Clinical Trials: Issues and Challenges
Tie-Hua Ng

Optimal Design for Nonlinear Response Models
Valerii V. Fedorov and Sergei L. Leonov

Patient-Reported Outcomes: Measurement, Implementation and Interpretation
Joseph C. Cappelleri, Kelly H. Zou, Andrew G. Bushmakin, Jose Ma. J. Alvir, Demissie Alemayehu, and Tara Symonds

Quantitative Evaluation of Safety in Drug Development: Design, Analysis and Reporting
Qi Jiang and H. Amy Xia

Randomized Clinical Trials of Nonpharmacological Treatments
Isabelle Boutron, Philippe Ravaud, and David Moher

Randomized Phase II Cancer Clinical Trials
Sin-Ho Jung

Sample Size Calculations for Clustered and Longitudinal Outcomes in Clinical Research
Chul Ahn, Moonseong Heo, and Song Zhang

Sample Size Calculations in Clinical Research, Second Edition
Shein-Chung Chow, Jun Shao and Hansheng Wang

Statistical Analysis of Human Growth and Development
Yin Bun Cheung

Statistical Design and Analysis of Stability Studies
Shein-Chung Chow

Statistical Evaluation of Diagnostic Performance: Topics in ROC Analysis
Kelly H. Zou, Aiyi Liu, Andriy Bandos, Lucila Ohno-Machado, and Howard Rockette

Statistical Methods for Clinical Trials
Mark X. Norleans

Statistical Methods in Drug Combination Studies
Wei Zhao and Harry Yang

Statistics in Drug Research: Methodologies and Recent Developments
Shein-Chung Chow and Jun Shao

Statistics in the Pharmaceutical Industry, Third Edition
Ralph Buncher and Jia-Yeong Tsay

Survival Analysis in Medicine and Genetics
Jialiang Li and Shuangge Ma

Theory of Drug Development
Eric B. Holmgren

Translational Medicine: Strategies and Statistical Methods
Dennis Cosmatos and Shein-Chung Chow

Chapman & Hall/CRC Biostatistics Series

Adaptive Designs for Sequential Treatment Allocation

Alessandro Baldi Antognini
University of Bologna, Italy

Alessandra Giovagnoli
University of Bologna, Italy

CRC Press
Taylor & Francis Group
Boca Raton London New York

CRC Press is an imprint of the
Taylor & Francis Group, an informa business
A CHAPMAN & HALL BOOK

CRC Press
Taylor & Francis Group
6000 Broken Sound Parkway NW, Suite 300
Boca Raton, FL 33487-2742

Printed on acid-free paper
Version Date: 20150225

International Standard Book Number-13: 978-1-4665-0575-9 (Hardback)

Visit the Taylor & Francis Web site at
http://www.taylorandfrancis.com

and the CRC Press Web site at
http://www.crcpress.com

This book is dedicated to all those teachers and colleagues who have made us love and respect mathematics.

Contents

List of Figures

List of Tables

Preface

This book addresses the issue of designing experiments for comparing two or more treatments, when the experiment is sequential and the experimenter wishes to make use of the information accrued along the way. This type of experimental design is called *adaptive*. The aim of the book is reviewing and reorganizing the existing results of adaptive design theory, with particular attention to its mathematical foundation. It is intended primarily as a research book. Our approach is essentially theoretical, highlighting the mathematical difficulties and the statistical properties of adaptive designs as regards statistical inference following the experiment. We feel that this approach is needed, since the choice of an experimental design cannot be made without a full understanding of its properties, and we hope that this book will complement part of the present day literature in which a large number of authors base their conclusions on simulations. Simulations are generally very useful, but not always sufficiently convincing, and in some cases they may be plainly misleading. Ours is a book mainly devoted to general results, so it does not address problems related only to particular applications. Specifically, it is *not* a book on clinical trials, although a large number of the designs we present are clearly inspired by clinical and pharmaceutical research, and the vast bibliography dedicated to this field. These designs are discussed, in particular, in Atkinson and Biswas' survey *Randomized Response-Adaptive Designs in Clinical Trials*, 2014; our motivations are different and we have chosen to dwell on general aspects more than on individual trials, so there is little overlap, and we think of our book as a complement to theirs. This book follows the lead of two fundamental works by W. F. Rosenberger and his coauthors (Hu and Rosenberger, *The Theory of Response-Adaptive Randomization in Clinical Trials*, 2006, and Rosenberger and Lachin, *Randomization in Clinical Trials: Theory and Practice*, 2002), to whom we are deeply indebted. We have updated several results and included new topics.

The first chapter introduces the terminology and the statistical models most commonly used in comparative experiments. We present target allocations of the treatments motivated by inferential considerations, and give new conditions for the convergence of a sequential experiment to a given target. A discussion of asymptotic inference plays a central role in the chapter. We also introduce a unifying definition (*Markovian Designs*) to describe a large class of adaptive designs that share interesting properties. We emphasize the role of randomization throughout, as an important tool to avoid several types of bias. The randomized adaptive designs that we present in the remaining chapters are grouped mainly according to methods of construction. In Chapter 2 we illustrate designs whose assignment rule takes into account past treatment allocations only, namely the renown biased coins and some urn ones. Then in Chapter 3 there come designs that make use of past data, too: sequential maximum likelihood designs and doubly-adaptive designs, with a further section on the topic of up-and-down experiments. In Chapters 4 and 5 we present multipurpose adaptive experiments, involving also utilitarian choices and/or ethical issues: these are classified according to whether the decision on how to proceed is based on a step-by-step compromise among the different objectives (Chapter 4), or an overall strategy that seeks a compound optimal allocation target (Chapter 5); the latter is a fairly novel approach, so the relative designs too are almost all new. The acquisition of covariate information (like prognostic factors, biomarkers) about the statistical units involved in the experiment is also of fundamental importance and should not be ignored in the design. In Chapter 6 adaptive experiments are revisited to include covariates and new adaptive methods for this context are presented. Throughout this book we make extensive reference to design optimality in the context of adaptive experiments, and the basic tools of optimal design theory used in this book are included as a separate appendix. There is also another appendix on Bayesian adaptive designs: this is a widely used methodology, and although our approach is frequentist, we regard this type of design conceptually very important, so much so as to deserve a full book devoted to them.

We are aware that several issues of great relevance for applied adaptive designs are not included or not fully discussed in this monograph, such as dose-ranging estimation, sample size re-estimation, adaptive hypotheses designs and seamless trial designs, to mention just a few. We do not feel that the theoretic study of some of these methodologies has reached sufficient maturity to be included in this monograph. Some other central topics are just hinted at, the most prominent of which is stopping rules (at the end of Chapter 1). This is due to the fact that there already exist outstanding books on this subject. Lastly, note that ours is a model-based approach, thus we do not include designing experiments for randomization-based inference.

We hope that researchers working in the area of adaptive designs will find this book a useful reference. Teachers of graduate-level courses on designs may find this useful since it includes a fair number of examples. The degree of mathematical sophistication required from the readers is a knowledge of elementary algebra, calculus and probability, and rudimentary notions of stochastic processes—in particular the theory of Markov chains. We have tried to avoid making explicit use of more advanced mathematical tools, such as Martingale theory, although some of the results we present (without proofs) are indeed based on such theories.

Acknowledgments

We are grateful to all our colleagues who showed their encouragement and gave us useful advice, in particular Anthony C. Atkinson, Rosemary Bailey, Barbara Bogacka, Steve Coad, Nancy Flournoy, Stefania Gubbiotti, Ludovico Piccinato, Giovanni Pistone, Luc Pronzato, Yosef Rinott, Bill Rosenberger, Piercesare Secchi, Henry Wynn, Maroussa Zagoraiou.

We are also deeply indebted to the referees who read early versions of the manuscript and helped us with their constructive remarks.

Dr. Giovagnoli wishes to express her thanks to The Newton Institute for the Mathematical Sciences, Cambridge, UK, for hospitality during the 2011 Design and Analysis of Experiments (DAE) Workshop, which marked the start of this work.

Introduction

The scientific paradigm for the study of phenomena with variable outcomes is one or more experiments followed by a statistical analysis of the observed data. A central role is played by the *model,* namely the mathematical scheme that describes how the phenomenon behaves. A large number of these experiments are for comparing the effects of different "treatments", possibly including one (or more) controls.

Planning the way in which the experiment will be performed, namely, the *experimental design,* is of fundamental importance. In this book we discuss experiments that are performed sequentially. Interest in sequential procedures can be traced back to sequential acceptance sampling by Wald (1947), with the possibility at each stage either to accept or to reject the sampled lot, or to continue the sampling. But the concepts and philosophy of sequential experimentation really took off in the 1960s, in particular with the well-known "play-the-winner" design (Zelen, 1969). Beginning with Efron (1971), sequential methods were employed in experiments in order to partially correct deviations from balanced treatment assignments. At the same time, a concern about balancing allocations among units with different characteristics led to the development of sequential covariate-adjustment rules by Zelen (1974) and Taves (1974).

Since then, experiments that take place in a sequential way have become increasingly common in different fields including educational testing, industrial engineering, clinical trials, etc. There are many reasons for wanting to carry out an experiment sequentially. In clinical trials, for instance, the main concern is monitoring the results to protect against adverse effects of the treatments. In industrial experiments, the intent is to increase efficiency and reduce costs. The correct design of these experiments poses challenging statistical problems and important advances have been made. This has developed into a new and important area of statistics called *Adaptive Designs.* The rigorous definition of an adaptive experiment is one performed in steps: at each step the decision about how to proceed next is made according to a pre-established rule that makes use of the information accrued along the way from the observed outcomes and/or statistical units. A useful introduction with real life examples is given by Rosenberger (1996).

Adaptive methods are attractive to experimenters: they look and often are more flexible, efficient, ethical and/or economical, and they seem to reflect actual practice in real life. Thus it is not surprising that statistical research on adaptive design theory and practice has advanced substantially over the past two decades. In the context of medical and pharmacological studies this is also due to strong encouragement from U.S. government agencies. Clearly the updating process of an experiment cannot take place in a haphazard manner, which could undermine the validity and integrity of the ensuing statistical analysis of the data: if some of the information acquired along the way is used to redirect the experiment itself, the common assumption of independent data may no longer hold. So the design of an adaptive experiment requires special care. U.S. health authorities have issued some important statements on statistical, clinical and regulatory aspects of adaptive designs in clinical research (CHMP, 2007; FDA, 2010). Following Sir Ronald Fisher, the father of experimental design theory, the allocations of the treatments to the units should generally include planned randomness as a protection against several forms of bias, in particular the selection bias arising from the investigators being able to guess the treatment allocations in advance (Blackwell and Hodges, 1957), the accidental bias due to the presence of potential confounders, the chronological bias related to potential time trends, etc. (Sverdlov and Rosenberger, 2013a). In planning clinical trials in particular, randomization is regarded as a must. If an experiment is adaptive, randomization means that the treatments are allocated to the next units by allocation probabilities that make use of the past experience.

There are several ways of designing an adaptive experiment for comparing two or more treatments, and most of them are reviewed in this book, with a focus on those that in our judgment are more relevant or more useful, or with a clearer justification. They have been classified according to what past information they make use of at each step, whether some or all the past allocations, whether just the most recent outcome or all the past outcomes, or whether they also use information about past and present statistical units. As to the methods of construction, there is a strong tradition in adaptive randomization to use urn models, but as we shall show, the theory of optimal designs plays an important role too; besides, new methods are often born out of combinations of existing ones. Moreover, it is not infrequent that an adaptive design is driven by the demand to approach a desirable target allocation, and we present theoretical results which ensure that this convergence takes place.

The aim of the experiment is clearly the motivating force behind its design, and adaptive designs are no exception. In a comparative experiment, the aim is usually to see whether the effects of the treatments differ, and by how much, in which case the experimenter's interest lies in maximizing the power of tests and the precision of estimates. But the experiment may also be partly utilitarian, i.e., aimed at maximizing the expected return or minimizing the expected loss; this may be due to an ethical or economic concern on maximizing the number of experimental units receiving the best treatments. There is a recent tendency to try to accommodate more than just one objective, typically mixing utility with statistical inference to get a compromise design that partly meets both demands, so special adaptive designs are also devised to serve more purposes.

Last but not least, a common request from practitioners is to know which adaptive design is the best for a particular problem. An attempt at choosing among several types of "biased coin" designs can be found in Atkinson (2014). Unfortunately there cannot be a single answer to this question, since the choice clearly depends on the purpose or purposes. Besides, since the actual realization of an adaptive design will be the outcome of chance and/or of the observed data, it is not even possible to establish in a clear-cut way of how good a design is on the basis of its real life implementations: had the outcome of the observations been different, the experiment would have evolved in a different way. Even the traditional rule "keep it simple!" has to be reconsidered in the light of the present available computer facilities that make even complicated adaptive designs relatively easy to put into practice. This justifies why the main emphasis of this book is on illustrating the theoretical properties of the designs.

1

Fundamentals and preliminary results

1.1 Contents of this chapter

In this first chapter we introduce the terminology, the main assumptions, and the statistical models most widely used in adaptive comparative experiments with v treatments. In particular the observed responses are assumed to behave according to one of the models belonging to the exponential family – see Section 1.3 – and we make the essential assumption that at each step, given the treatment assigned to the experimental unit, the response is independent of the other observations. The role of the ensuing Fisher information in an adaptive design setting is highlighted in Section 1.4.

In Section 1.5 there is a discussion of the type of inferential approach to be adopted, whether we should condition on the experimental design regardless of the fact that it has been achieved as a realization of a sequential process or whether, on the contrary, inference should be unconditional, as argued by Rosenberger and Lachin (2002). This essentially depends on whether the design is of the allocation-adaptive type, i.e., the randomization mechanism for the choice of the next treatment is a function of the past allocations only, or response-adaptive, i.e., dependent on past data as well.

In Section 1.6 we discuss the meaning of inferential optimality for an adaptive design, and Section 1.7 presents some treatment allocations, i.e., *targets*, motivated by the classical theory of Optimal Designs. An adaptive design is defined to be asymptotically optimal if it converges to an optimal target. Section 1.8 contains several conditions for the convergence of an adaptive design to a desired target and the asymptotic properties of the maximum likelihood estimators, followed by some illustrative examples in Section 1.9 related to a simple type of experiment: the Sequential Maximum Likelihood design. In Section 1.8 we also give the result that in most common cases a treatment allocation which is asymptotically optimal for conditional inference is also optimal when the inference is unconditional.

Section 1.10 is dedicated to the study of the properties of a large class of adaptive designs with a Markovian-type characterization, again followed by examples: Biased Coins, Play-the-Winner, Up-and-Down (Section 1.11). Section 1.12 deals with rules for stopping the experiment on the basis of the accrued data; by their very nature these rules are always adaptive.

Lastly, Section 1.13 tackles the implementation of adaptive designs in comparative experiments; for instance, a practical problem is when the responses are delayed, so that the decision about the next treatment assignment is to be made before the outcomes of the most recent ones are observed. There is also a brief hint at the case of missing data. The controversial issue of simulation is discussed in Section 1.14.

1.2 Some notation

We start this chapter by introducing some basic notation. Comparative experiments of the sequential type are the object of our study. We wish to compare v treatments $T_1, \ldots, T_v$: each unit of our sample will be assigned one of the treatments and a scalar response Y will be observed. Typically, the outcome Y will depend, as well as on the treatment, on some characteristics of the statistical unit, generally referred to as covariates or block effects. We will deal with covariates in Chapter 6, but for the time being we are not going to take them into account.

We also suppose that the statistical units enter the trial one after the other, and at each step only one treatment is assigned. At step i, let $\boldsymbol{\delta}_i = (\delta_{1i}, \ldots, \delta_{vi})^t$ denote the allocation vector by $\delta_{ji} = 1$ if unit i is allocated to treatment T_j, and 0 otherwise; clearly $\sum_{j=1}^{v} \delta_{ji} = 1$. We write $\delta^{(n)} = \{\boldsymbol{\delta}_1, \ldots, \boldsymbol{\delta}_n\}$ for the allocation sequence after n steps, and $Y^{(n)} = \{Y_1, \ldots, Y_n\}$ for the sequence of responses up to n; both $\delta^{(0)}$ and $Y^{(0)}$ will denote the empty set. Furthermore, let $N_{jn} = \sum_{k=1}^{n} \delta_{jk}$ and $\pi_{jn} = n^{-1} N_{jn}$ denote the number and the proportion of assignments of treatment j, respectively, and write $\boldsymbol{N}_n = (N_{1n}, \ldots, N_{vn})^t$ and $\boldsymbol{\pi}_n = (\pi_{1n}, \ldots, \pi_{vn})^t$.

For specific problems the notation introduced so far appears unduly complex: oftentimes the number of treatments to be compared is just two, and we shall use A and B instead of T_1 and T_2. With just two treatments there is no need to resort to an allocation vector $\boldsymbol{\delta}_i = (\delta_{1i}, \delta_{2i})^t$, since $\delta_{2i} = 1 - \delta_{1i}$, so it suffices to use δ_i as the indicator for treatment A at stage i, and similarly π_n will be the proportion of allocations to A after n steps.

The treatment allocation rule may be deterministic or stochastic: a general way of representing it consists in the sequence given by the allocation probability of each treatment at stage 1 and the conditional probabilities of assigning the treatment given the past allocations and observations at every subsequent stage $i \geq 2$:

$$\Pr(\delta_{j1} = 1) \quad \text{and} \quad \Pr\left(\delta_{ji} = 1 | \delta^{(i-1)}, Y^{(i-1)}\right), \qquad j = 1, \ldots, v. \tag{1.1}$$

We write the sequence of all these probabilities as

$$\left\{\Re\left(\boldsymbol{\delta}_i \mid \delta^{(i-1)}, Y^{(i-1)}\right)\right\}_{i \geq 1}. \tag{1.2}$$

Because of the dependence of (1.2) on the past allocations and observations, the experimental design will be a stochastic process, whose realization is the sequence of treatment assignments that actually take place in the experiment. The treatment allocations behave like data, and the experimental information arising from n observations will be described by the natural history of the experiment up to step n, namely the sequence $\Im_n = \{(\boldsymbol{\delta}_1, Y_1), \ldots, (\boldsymbol{\delta}_n, Y_n)\}$.

Another useful concept related to the experiment is that of a *statistic*. For a given n, a statistic is a function of the data up to step n, i.e., $S_n = s(\boldsymbol{\delta}_1, Y_1, \ldots, \boldsymbol{\delta}_n, Y_n)$. A typical statistic is $n^{-1}\sum_{i=1}^{n} \delta_{ji} Y_i$, the average outcome on treatment j in the first n observations. A special case is when the statistic is a function of just the design points: we will refer to it as a *design statistic* $S_n^d = s^d(\boldsymbol{\delta}_1, \ldots, \boldsymbol{\delta}_n)$. For instance $N_{jn} = \sum_{k=1}^{n} \delta_{jk}$, the number of times treatment j is assigned in the first n runs, is a design statistic. When the design is sequential, we deal with sequences $\{S_n\}_{n\in\mathbb{N}}$ of statistics. A design statistic sequence will be said to *generate* the design when it contains all the information on the experiment: in other words, given $\{s_n^d\}_{n\in\mathbb{N}}$ it is possible to retrieve the sequence of the design points $\{\boldsymbol{\delta}_n\}_{n\in\mathbb{N}}$. More in general, at each step n we would usually consider a vector of statistics, for example

$$\left(\frac{N_{1n}}{n}, \frac{1}{n}\sum_{i=1}^{n} \delta_{1i} Y_i, \frac{N_{2n}}{n}, \frac{1}{n}\sum_{i=1}^{n} \delta_{2i} Y_i\right).$$

In sequential adaptive designs, usually the dependence of the assignments on the past history is obtained defining the allocation probabilities (1.1) at step n to be functions of a vector of statistics related to the experiment.

In the next chapters we shall deal with the two separate cases of whether the allocation rule (1.1) is of the simpler form

$$\left\{\Pr\left(\delta_{ji} = 1 \mid \delta^{(i-1)}\right), j = 1, \ldots, v\right\}$$

or also dependent on the observations; in other words, whether one modifies the experiment along the way on the basis of just the past allocations or of the observed responses too. For the former case, a suggested terminology is *allocation-adaptive* design. For the latter, the standard terminology is *response-adaptive*, but some authors also use *response-driven* or *stage-wise data-dependent* designs, or similar expressions; see, for instance, the discussion in Rosenberger and Lachin (2002). A word of warning: care should be paid when meeting with the expression *response-adaptive randomization*. In this book it means any randomization device that at each step depends on the accrued data. In the context of clinical trials, however, it often implies a process to allocate more patients to some treatments that appear more promising than the others (see Coad (2008)).

1.3 Statistical models

The great majority of models used to describe the behaviour of the responses are parametric ones, with some parameters being of interest for inference and others being nuisance parameters. We denote by $\mathcal{L}(Y_1, \gamma|\boldsymbol{\delta}_1)$ and $\{\mathcal{L}(Y_i, \gamma|\delta^{(i)}, Y^{(i-1)})\}$ the probability laws of the responses at steps 1 and $i \geq 2$ respectively, which we assume to depend on a vector of unknown parameters $\gamma \in \Omega$, where Ω is an open convex subset of $\mathbb{R}^q$. It is often the case that $\gamma = (\theta_1, \ldots, \theta_r; \phi_1, \ldots, \phi_s)^t$, with $\theta_h \in \mathbb{R}$ $(h = 1, \ldots, r)$ parameters of interest and $\phi_k \in \mathbb{R}^+$ $(k = 1, \ldots, s)$ nuisance parameters. The most frequent cases are $r = s = v$ or $r = v,\ s = 1$.

The following is often assumed to hold true:

Condition 1 *Conditionally on the allocations, the observations are independent. More precisely,*

$$\mathcal{L}(Y_i; \gamma|\delta^{(i)}, Y^{(i-1)}) = \mathcal{L}(Y_i; \gamma|\boldsymbol{\delta}_i), \qquad \forall i \geq 1. \tag{1.3}$$

In other words, the only interdependence among the responses arises from the treatment assignments.

Further assumptions are:

Condition 2 *For all $i \geq 1$, $\mathcal{L}(Y_i, \gamma|\boldsymbol{\delta}_i)$ satisfies the usual Rao–Cramer regularity conditions, to be found for instance in Cox and Hinkley (1974).*

Condition 3 *For all $i \geq 1$, the conditional distribution $\Re\left(\boldsymbol{\delta}_{i+1}|\delta^{(i)}, Y^{(i)}\right)$ of the design point $\boldsymbol{\delta}_{i+1}$ does not depend on γ.*

A very general model, particularly useful in practice, is described by the *regular exponential family*: for any $j = 1, \ldots, v$, the observations relative to treatment j are assumed to be identically distributed for all $i \geq 1$, with probability or density of the form

$$f_j(y) = \exp\left\{\phi_j^{-1}[a(\theta_j)y - b(\theta_j)] + c(y, \phi_j)\right\}, \quad \forall j = 1, \ldots, v, \tag{1.4}$$

with $a(\cdot)$ and $b(\cdot)$ twice continuously differentiable functions.

Special cases of particular relevance for applications are:

1. **Bernoulli model**

$$\begin{aligned} \Pr(Y_i = y \mid \delta_{ji} = 1) &= p_j^y(1 - p_j)^{1-y} \\ &= \exp\left\{y \log\left(\frac{p_j}{1 - p_j}\right) + \log(1 - p_j)\right\}, \end{aligned} \tag{1.5}$$

with $y \in \{0; 1\}$ and $p_j \in (0; 1)$;

2. **Logit model**, obtained from (1.5) by letting $\eta_j = \log[p_j/(1 - p_j)]$

$$\Pr(Y_i = y \mid \delta_{ji} = 1) = \exp\{y\eta_j - \log(1 + e^{\eta_j})\}; \tag{1.6}$$

3. **Normal model**

$$f_j(y) = \frac{1}{\sqrt{2\pi\sigma_j^2}} \exp\left\{-\frac{(y-\mu_j)^2}{2\sigma_j^2}\right\} \tag{1.7}$$

$$= \exp\left\{\left(\sigma_j^2\right)^{-1}\left(\mu_j y - \frac{\mu_j^2}{2}\right) - \frac{y^2}{2\sigma_j^2} - \frac{1}{2}\log\left(2\pi\sigma_j^2\right)\right\},$$

with $y \in \mathbb{R}$, $\mu_j \in \mathbb{R}$ and $\sigma_j^2 \in \mathbb{R}^+$; the case of different σ_j^2 is known as the *heteroscedastic* model, while it is the *homoscedastic* model if all the σ_j^2 are equal:

$$f_j(y) = \frac{1}{\sqrt{2\pi\sigma^2}} \exp\left\{-\frac{(y-\mu_j)^2}{2\sigma^2}\right\} \tag{1.8}$$

$$= \exp\left\{\left(\sigma^2\right)^{-1}\left(\mu_j y - \frac{\mu_j^2}{2}\right) - \frac{y^2}{2\sigma^2} - \frac{\log\left(2\pi\sigma^2\right)}{2}\right\}; \tag{1.9}$$

4. **Exponential model**

$$f_j(y) = \lambda_j \exp\{-\lambda_j y\} = \exp\{-\lambda_j y + \log\lambda_j\}, \tag{1.10}$$

with $y \in \mathbb{R}^+$ and $\lambda_j \in \mathbb{R}^+$.

1.4 The likelihood and Fisher's information

For a sample of size n, the conditional independence assumption (1.3) leads to the following expression for the likelihood of the vector $\boldsymbol{\gamma}$:

$$L_n\left(\delta^{(n)}, y^{(n)}\right) = \prod_{i=1}^{n} \mathcal{L}\left(y_i, \boldsymbol{\gamma} \mid \boldsymbol{\delta}_i\right) \times \prod_{i=1}^{n} \Re\left(\boldsymbol{\delta}_i \mid \delta^{(i-1)}, y^{(i-1)}\right). \tag{1.11}$$

The product

$$\prod_{i=1}^{n} \Re\left(\boldsymbol{\delta}_i \mid \delta^{(i-1)}, y^{(i-1)}\right)$$

does not depend on the unknown parameters of the model, so the Maximum Likelihood Estimators of $\boldsymbol{\gamma}$ after n observations are

$$\hat{\boldsymbol{\gamma}}_n = \arg\max_{\boldsymbol{\gamma}\in\Omega} \prod_{i=1}^{n} \mathcal{L}(Y_i; \boldsymbol{\gamma} \mid \boldsymbol{\delta}_i) \tag{1.12}$$

for a sequential design too. However, the distribution of the MLEs will not be the same as in the non-sequential case and in general will depend on the design. This inferential problem is sometimes overlooked, as McCullagh (1981) was among the first to point out.

From (1.11) we obtain the expression for the Fisher information matrix $\mathbf{I}\left(\gamma \mid \delta^{(n)}\right)$ of the parameter vector γ conditional on the design sequence $\delta^{(n)}$. The matrix $\mathbf{M}\left(\gamma \mid \delta^{(n)}\right)$:

$$\mathbf{M}\left(\gamma \mid \delta^{(n)}\right) = n^{-1}\mathbf{I}\left(\gamma \mid \delta^{(n)}\right) = \frac{1}{n}\sum_{i=1}^{n}\left(E\left[\frac{-\partial^2 \log \mathcal{L}(Y_i, \gamma \mid \boldsymbol{\delta}_i)}{\partial\gamma_h \partial\gamma_k} \mid \boldsymbol{\delta}_i\right]\right)_{hk} \tag{1.13}$$

is usually referred to as the *normalized* Fisher information. As is well known, under Conditions 1-3 of Section 1.3, expression (1.13) is the inverse of the asymptotic variance-covariance matrix of the MLEs conditional on the design. The expectations $E[\cdot]$ inside the brackets of (1.13) are calculated with respect to the conditional model $\mathcal{L}\left(Y_i; \gamma \mid \boldsymbol{\delta}_i\right)$.

The normalized unconditional Fisher information is:

$$\mathbf{M}(\gamma) = \frac{1}{n}\sum_{i=1}^{n} E\left[E\left(\frac{-\partial^2 \log L(\gamma \mid \boldsymbol{\delta}_i, Y_i)}{\partial\gamma_h \partial\gamma_k} \mid \boldsymbol{\delta}_i\right)\right]_{hk}, \tag{1.14}$$

where now the outer bracket expectation refers to the corresponding marginal distribution of the ith design allocation $\boldsymbol{\delta}_i$.

It is worth stressing that, unlike (1.13), matrix (1.14)

- is not random,
- depends on the generating rule of the design through the marginal distributions of the $\boldsymbol{\delta}_i$'s.

In the context of unconditional inference, the unconditional Fisher information (1.14) may be a useful tool, but the exact distribution of the design sequence $\delta^{(n)}$ is likely to be unattainable.

We now apply the above discussion to calculating Fisher's information for models belonging to the exponential family (1.4). Discarding the information on the nuisance vector $\boldsymbol{\phi} = (\phi_1, \ldots, \phi_v)^t$, after n steps the normalized Fisher information conditional on the design associated with $\boldsymbol{\theta} = (\theta_1, \ldots, \theta_v)$ is a $v \times v$ diagonal matrix which depends on $\delta^{(n)}$ only through the current vector $\boldsymbol{\pi}_n$ of allocations, namely

$$\mathbf{M}(\boldsymbol{\theta}|\boldsymbol{\pi}_n) = \text{diag}\left(\pi_{jn}\, s(\theta_j; \phi_j)\right)_{j=1,\ldots,v} \tag{1.15}$$

where $s(\theta_j; \phi_j)$ is the *score* associated with θ_j

$$s(\theta_j; \phi_j) = \phi_j^{-1}\left[b''(\theta_j) - \frac{b'(\theta_j)}{a'(\theta_j)}\, a''(\theta_j)\right], \qquad j = 1, \ldots, v. \tag{1.16}$$

Note that:

i) there is no direct dependence of the information matrix (1.15) on n;

ii) since every $s(\theta_j;\phi_j)$ is a continuous function of the parameters, $\mathbf{M}(\boldsymbol{\theta}|\boldsymbol{\pi}_n)$ too is a continuous function of $\boldsymbol{\theta}$, $\boldsymbol{\phi}$ and $\boldsymbol{\pi}_n$;

iii) for a fixed sample size n the normalized conditional Fisher information (1.15) is the same, whether the design is sequential or not.

If, without loss of generality, we assume the exponential family (1.4) parameterized as follows:

$$\theta_j = E[Y_i|\delta_{ji}=1], \qquad \forall j=1,2,\ldots,v, \quad i\geq 1, \tag{1.17}$$

then the MLEs $\hat{\boldsymbol{\theta}}_n = (\hat{\theta}_{1n}, \hat{\theta}_{2n}, \ldots, \hat{\theta}_{vn})^t$ of $\boldsymbol{\theta}$ are the sample means:

$$\hat{\theta}_{jn} = \frac{\sum_{i=1}^{n} \delta_{ji} Y_i}{N_{jn}}, \qquad j=1,2,\ldots,v \tag{1.18}$$

and at each step n, the normalized conditional Fisher information becomes

$$\mathbf{M}(\boldsymbol{\theta} \mid \boldsymbol{\pi}_n) = \text{diag}\left(\frac{\pi_{1n}}{Var[Y_i|\delta_{1i}=1]}; \ldots; \frac{\pi_{vn}}{Var[Y_i|\delta_{vi}=1]}\right). \tag{1.19}$$

Expression (1.19) may depend on the nuisance parameters $\boldsymbol{\phi}$ too.

For the examples of Section 1.3 the normalized conditional Fisher information (1.15) is, respectively:

1. **Bernoulli model**

$$\mathbf{M}(p_1,\ldots,p_v \mid \boldsymbol{\pi}_n) = \text{diag}\left(\frac{\pi_{jn}}{p_j(1-p_j)}\right)_{j=1,\ldots,v}; \tag{1.20}$$

2. **Logit model**

$$\mathbf{M}(\eta_1,\ldots,\eta_v \mid \boldsymbol{\pi}_n) = \text{diag}\left(\pi_{jn}\frac{e^{\eta_j}}{(1+e^{\eta_j})^2}\right)_{j=1,\ldots,v}; \tag{1.21}$$

3. **Normal model**

$$\mathbf{M}(\mu_1,\ldots,\mu_v \mid \boldsymbol{\pi}_n) = \text{diag}\left(\frac{\pi_{jn}}{\sigma_j^2}\right)_{j=1,\ldots,v}; \tag{1.22}$$

4. **Exponential model**

$$\mathbf{M}(\lambda_1,\ldots,\lambda_v \mid \boldsymbol{\pi}_n) = \text{diag}\left(\lambda_j^2 \pi_{jn}\right)_{j=1,\ldots,v}. \tag{1.23}$$

The **unconditional** normalized Fisher information for $\boldsymbol{\theta}$ is

$$\mathbf{M}(\boldsymbol{\theta}) = E\left[\mathbf{M}(\boldsymbol{\theta} \mid \boldsymbol{\pi}_n)\right], \tag{1.24}$$

where the expected value is taken with respect to the distribution of the random vector $\boldsymbol{\pi}_n$ of treatment proportions. This implies that in expressions (1.20), (1.21), (1.22) and (1.23) above, π_{jn} is replaced by $E[\pi_{jn}]$ (for $j=1,\ldots,v$).

1.5 Inference: Conditional on the design or unconditional?

When the experiment is sequential, the potentially random nature of the experimental design may pose some problems for the statistical analysis of the experimental data. The question of the correct inferential paradigm after a sequential experiment was first posed by Silvey (1980). Later, Rosenberger and Lachin (2002) (Chapter 11) have dealt with the question of response-adaptive design in depth and pointed out the inferential pitfalls.

The prevailing viewpoint in practical applications is to draw inferences conditionally on the design; in other words the same inferential methods are applied, whether or not the sample size and the sequence of the design points are predetermined. The present authors share the opinion that for sequential designs it does make a difference whether or not the allocation rule is response-adaptive. An allocation-adaptive design, i.e., such that the design points do not depend on previous observations, is non-informative about the unknown parameter $\boldsymbol{\theta}$. The design as a whole can be thought of as an extended *ancillary statistic* (see Cox (2006)): then a conditional inference approach is justified (see for instance Lindsey (1996)).

On the other hand, when the allocation rule is response-adaptive, the design realization is in itself informative about $\boldsymbol{\theta}$ and conditional inference entails a partial loss of information. Inference should be unconditional, namely should take into account the randomness of the design as well. This point of view can be found for instance in Rosenberger and Lachin (2002).

It would not escape even the most absent-minded reader that unconditional inference is mathematically very complex. As already pointed out, the Maximum Likelihood estimators are the same as for non-adaptive designs, but not their distribution. The estimators will usually be biased, and the confidence intervals based on the usual pivots will not have the correct coverage probability; the distribution of common statistics for testing treatment equality under the alternative hypothesis will also be affected. Getting exact results for a given finite sample size n in most cases appears to be an impossible task.

A way out is to use approximations based on asymptotic results, when available. A notable exception is the work of Woodroofe and Coad (1996) and Coad and Woodroofe (2005), who build confidence intervals using finite sample approximations based on Edgeworth expansions.

1.6 Inferential optimality of an adaptive design

In the non-sequential case, some common methods for choosing the best design are rooted in Optimal Design theory (see Appendix A): the key idea is to choose a criterion that measures *loss* as a function of the variance-covariance of the estimators or a function of the information matrix. We need to clarify what we mean by designs that are optimal for treatment comparison when the design points are obtained in a sequence. Suppose we stop observing after n steps, with n chosen in advance; we get the conditional information matrix (1.13). If we are going to infer conditionally on the design, this is the information we want to optimize with respect to a given criterion Φ. Thus an optimal design for estimating the treatments will be any sequence $\delta^{(n)*}$ such that

$$\delta^{(n)*} = \arg\min \Phi\left(\mathbf{M}\left(\boldsymbol{\theta} \mid \delta^{(n)}\right)\right), \qquad \forall \boldsymbol{\theta} \in \Theta.$$

As regards estimating treatments unconditionally, arguing along similar lines leads to defining optimal designs as the ones that minimize the unconditional variance-covariance matrix of the estimators of the parameters of interest with respect to a suitable criterion. It is more common, however, to try and optimize the unconditional information (1.14), namely to look for an allocation rule that generates a design process $\delta^{(n)**}$ such that

$$\delta^{(n)**} = \arg\min \Phi\left(E_{\delta^{(n)}}\left[\mathbf{M}\left(\boldsymbol{\theta} \mid \delta^{(n)}\right)\right]\right), \qquad \forall \boldsymbol{\theta} \in \Theta,$$

where we are minimizing with respect to the distribution of $\delta^{(n)}$. The underlying assumption is that (1.14) is, at least approximately, proportional to the inverse of the variance-covariance of the estimators.

When the purpose of the experiment is to test a specific statistical hypothesis on the treatment effects, optimality will consist in maximizing the power of the test uniformly over the unknown parameters. A similar argument as above holds: for sequential experiments, the power of the test is random, due to the randomness of the design or the dependence on the data. When inference is unconditional, following a response-adaptive design, our approach is to choose designs that maximize the expected power. For finite n, in general this will be unfeasible to compute so other approaches have been considered, as will be shown in more detail in Section 1.7.

1.7 Most informative targets

In comparative experiments with v treatments, we shall refer to all the desirable treatment allocation proportions $\boldsymbol{\pi} = (\pi_1, \ldots, \pi_v)^t$ as "targets". The target $\boldsymbol{\pi}$ can be either an actual desired proportion of assignments to $T_1, \ldots, T_v$ out of a total of n observations, or a limit to which the allocation proportions should ideally converge as n increases.

A special case is when targets are obtained from Optimal Design theory. When inference is conditional on the design, optimal targets for estimating the parameters are obtained applying one of the optimality criteria of Appendix A to the conditional variance-covariance matrix of the estimates, or the conditional information matrix; see Appendix A. Since the observations are assumed to be independent conditionally on the treatment, they are exchangeable, namely any permutation of their order does not alter the Fisher information matrix and the optimal design is a vector of proportions of the total sample size, one for each treatment, which optimizes the chosen criterion.

Example 1.1 *Let A and B be the two treatments and suppose that the responses belong to the exponential family (1.4). We assume the exponential family to be parameterized as in (1.17), namely let*

$$\theta_A = E[Y_i \mid \delta_i = 1] \quad \text{and} \quad \theta_B = E[Y_i \mid \delta_i = 0]$$

be the treatment effects. Conditionally on the treatment assignment, the observations are independent and identically distributed (iid), so we can also write

$$Var[Y_A] = Var[Y_i \mid \delta_i = 1] \quad \text{and} \quad Var[Y_B] = Var[Y_i \mid \delta_i = 0].$$

For the one-parameter models in the exponential family (such as Bernoulli, Exponential, etc...), the treatment responses are stochastically ordered on the basis of their effects, namely if $\theta_A \geq \theta_B$ then $\mathrm{F}_{Y_A}(y) \leq \mathrm{F}_{Y_B}(y)$ for all y, where $\mathrm{F}_Y(y)$ denotes the cumulative distribution function (cdf) of the random variable Y. The same holds true for the exponential family models with parameters $\gamma_A = (\theta_A, \phi)$ and $\gamma_B = (\theta_B, \phi)$, where the common ϕ is a nuisance; this clearly includes the normal homoscedastic case.

Expression (1.19) now becomes

$$\mathbf{M}(\theta_A; \theta_B \mid \pi_n) = diag\left(\frac{\pi_n}{Var[Y_A]}; \frac{1-\pi_n}{Var[Y_B]}\right) \tag{1.25}$$

and the optimal inferential target with respect to an inferential criterion Φ is the allocation

$$\pi_{\mathcal{I}}^* = \arg \min_{\pi \in [0;1]} \Phi\left[\mathbf{M}^{-1}(\theta_A; \theta_B \mid \pi)\right]. \tag{1.26}$$

We underline that target $\pi_{\mathcal{I}}^*$ will in general depend on the unknown model parameters, not only the treatment effects but also the nuisances, if present.

When interest is in the joint estimation of the unknown treatment effects, the D-optimality Φ_D is usually applied, namely

$$\Phi_D(\pi) = \det\left[\mathbf{M}^{-1}(\theta_A; \theta_B \mid \pi)\right] = \frac{Var[Y_A] \cdot Var[Y_B]}{\pi(1-\pi)}, \tag{1.27}$$

and criterion (1.27) is always minimized when the two treatment groups are balanced. For normal responses $N(\mu_j; \sigma_j^2)$ $(j = A, B)$, (1.27) becomes

$$\Phi_D(\pi) = \Phi_D[\mathbf{M}^{-1}(\mu_A; \mu_B \mid \pi)] = \frac{\sigma_A^2 \sigma_B^2}{\pi(1-\pi)}, \tag{1.28}$$

while in the case of binary outcomes $Be(p_j)$ $(j = A, B)$ we have

$$\Phi_D(\pi) = \Phi_D[\mathbf{M}^{-1}(p_A; p_B \mid \pi)] = \frac{p_A q_A p_B q_B}{\pi(1-\pi)}. \tag{1.29}$$

If the experimental aim is to estimate the difference $\theta_A - \theta_B$, the A-optimality criterion

$$\Phi_A(\pi) = tr[\mathbf{M}^{-1}(\theta_A; \theta_B \mid \pi)] = \frac{Var[Y_A]}{\pi} + \frac{Var[Y_B]}{1-\pi} \quad (1.30)$$

is proportional to the variance of the estimated treatment difference, and it is minimized by the well-known Neyman allocation:

$$\pi_N^* = \frac{\sqrt{Var[Y_A]}}{\sqrt{Var[Y_A]} + \sqrt{Var[Y_B]}}.$$

In the context of binary responses, other inferentially optimal targets are obtained considering other criteria like the non-centrality parameter of the non-central chi-squared distribution with 1 degree of freedom of the Wald test statistic (Tymofyeyev et al., 2007).

Optimal allocation proportions for treatment comparison for some common linear and non-linear models with respect to most of the criteria mentioned above are listed for instance in Sverdlov and Rosenberger (2013a). Table 1.1 gives some examples for the exponential family (1.4).

TABLE 1.1: Some optimal targets for the exponential family

Parametric models	**Optimality criteria** *D*-	*A*-	*E*-
Normal (μ_j, σ_j)	$\frac{1}{v}$	$\frac{\sigma_j}{\sum_{s=1}^{v} \sigma_s}$	$\frac{\sigma_j^2}{\sum_{s=1}^{v} \sigma_s^2}$
Binary (p_j)	$\frac{1}{v}$	$\frac{\sqrt{p_j(1-p_j)}}{\sum_{s=1}^{v} \sqrt{p_s(1-p_s)}}$	$\frac{p_j(1-p_j)}{\sum_{s=1}^{v} p_s(1-p_s)}$
Logit (η_j)	$\frac{1}{v}$	$\frac{\frac{1+e^{\eta_j}}{\sqrt{e^{\eta_j}}}}{\sum_{s=1}^{v} \frac{1+e^{\eta_s}}{\sqrt{e^{\eta_s}}}}$	$\frac{\frac{\left(1+e^{\eta_j}\right)^2}{e^{\eta_j}}}{\sum_{s=1}^{v} \frac{(1+e^{\eta_s})^2}{e^{\eta_s}}}$
Exponential $(\theta_j = \lambda_j^{-1})$	$\frac{1}{v}$	$\frac{\theta_j}{\sum_{s=1}^{v} \theta_s}$	$\frac{\theta_j^2}{\sum_{s=1}^{v} \theta_s^2}$

Remark 1.1 *The balanced design, namely $\pi_j = v^{-1}$ for all $j = 1, \ldots, v$, is D-optimal for all the models of Table 1.1 and is optimal with respect to all three criteria for the normal homoscedastic model, as is evident from Appendix A.*

For response-adaptive designs and unconditional inference, the targets of Table 1.1 represent the optimal values of $E[\pi_{jn}]$ for every $j = 1, \ldots, v$.

As for tests, the most common case is when there are two treatments, A and B, and the null hypothesis is equality of the mean effects $\theta_j = E[Y_i \mid \delta_{ji} = 1]$ for $j = A, B$ ($i \geq 1$):

$$H_0: \quad \theta_A = \theta_B$$

versus the two-sided alternative $\theta_A \neq \theta_B$. If the test is Wald's (asymptotically equivalent to the likelihood-ratio test or the score test), in a conditional inference approach we obtain the same criterion as A-optimality, giving Neyman's allocation – namely allocation proportional to the standard deviation of the response conditional on the treatment – as the optimal target (see examples in Table 1.1).

In an unconditional inference context, we suggest to maximize the expected power but not all authors follow this approach. For instance, for the binary model Hu and Rosenberger (2003) use a normal approximation for the distribution of the test statistic and show that the asymptotic power is a decreasing function of the non-centrality parameter of the chi-squared distribution with 1 degree of freedom. Using a Taylor expansion, they also show that for a response-adaptive design the power is an increasing function of the design variability, namely the variance of the allocation proportions. Hence their viewpoint is that one can gauge whether a design has asymptotically best power by whether its asymptotic variance attains its minimum (Hu et al., 2006; Hu and Rosenberger, 2006). This leads to the definition of an *asymptotically best* design, which will be further discussed in Chapter 3.

However, using Large Deviation approximation, other authors (Azriel et al., 2012) show that for binary responses with two treatments the optimal design is close (but not identical) to the balanced design, and different from the Neyman allocation target to which the CLT approximation leads. This is due to the fact that the rate of convergence of the CLT is slow, and the normal distribution is not suitable for approximating the tails of the distribution of interest.

1.8 Asymptotic inference

In this section we deal with large sample properties of the design and the estimators of the parameters.

1.8.1 Convergence to a target

When the desired proportions of assignments do not depend on the sample size n, as the ones in Section 1.7, they can be regarded as desirable targets which the actual allocation proportion in the experiment should aim at approaching with probability one.

Definition 1.1 *We say that a sequential design converges to a target $\pi^0 = \pi^0(\gamma)$ if*

$$\lim_{n\to\infty} \frac{N_{jn}}{n} = \pi_j^0(\gamma) \quad \textit{almost surely} \quad \forall \gamma \in \Omega, \quad \textit{for all } j = 1, \ldots, v. \tag{1.31}$$

This will be the case for most of the examples discussed in the rest of this book. We shall indicate this convergence by $\lim_{n\to\infty} \boldsymbol{\pi}_n = \boldsymbol{\pi}^0 \; a.s.$

We now give a theoretical result that helps establish convergence in several practical cases. The proof can be found in Baldi Antognini and Giovagnoli (2006).

Theorem 1.1 *A sequential design converges to* $\boldsymbol{\pi}^0(\gamma)$ *if and only if*

$$\lim_{n\to\infty} \frac{1}{n}\sum_{i=1}^{n} P\left(\delta_{j,i+1} = 1 \mid \delta^{(i)}, Y^{(i)}\right) = \pi_j^0(\gamma) \quad \forall \gamma \in \Omega, \quad \forall j = 1, \ldots, v. \tag{1.32}$$

The expression on the left hand side of (1.32) is the Cesáro mean of the sequence of allocation probabilities, which is well-known to converge if the sequence converges, but not vice versa.

For the case of just two treatments A and B, there is another useful convergence result whose proof is given in Baldi Antognini and Zagoraiou (2015). Starting with n_0 observations on each treatment, assume that an initial non-trivial parameter estimation is derived. Then, at each step $n \geq 2n_0$, let $\widehat{\gamma}_n$ be an estimator of the parameter γ based on the first n observations, which is consistent in the iid case.

Theorem 1.2 *Let the allocation rule be of the form*

$$\Pr(\delta_{n+1} = 1 \mid \Im_n) = \varphi\left(\pi_n\,; \widehat{\gamma}_n\right), \qquad \text{for all } n \geq 2n_0, \tag{1.33}$$

where the function $\varphi(x, \mathbf{y}) : [0;1] \times \mathbb{R}^q \to [0;1]$ *is decreasing in* x*. If there exists a continuous function* $t(\mathbf{y}) : \mathbb{R}^q \to [0;1]$ *(which can be shown to be unique) such that for all* $\mathbf{y} \in \mathbb{R}^q$

$$\varphi(x, \mathbf{y}) \geq t(\mathbf{y}) \quad \forall x < t(\mathbf{y}) \quad \text{and} \quad \varphi(x, \mathbf{y}) \leq t(\mathbf{y}) \quad \forall x > t(\mathbf{y}),$$

then $t(\gamma) \neq 0, 1$ *and* $\lim_{n\to\infty} \pi_n = t(\gamma) \quad a.s. \quad \forall \gamma.$

Theorems 1.1 and 1.2 play a complementary role: by applying either of them it is often possible to prove the convergence of a given sequential design.

1.8.2 Asymptotic properties of maximum likelihood estimators

As already pointed out in Section 1.4, whether or not the sequential design is adaptive, the maximum likelihood estimators (MLEs) are the same as if the observed design points and the sample size were predetermined. It is important to stress again, however, that the distribution of the MLEs in general is not the same as when the observations are iid. Conditions under which the MLEs retain the strong consistency and asymptotic normality properties in the adaptive case too have been given by several authors (Wu, 1985; Chaudhuri and Mykland, 1993; Rosenberger et al., 1997). In actual practice the problem lies exactly in the possibility of checking whether or not such conditions are satisfied in a specific instance. In particular, Melfi and Page

(2000) show that estimators which are strongly consistent when the observations are iid will preserve this property under any sequential randomized procedure such that

$$\lim_{n\to\infty} N_{jn} = \infty \quad a.s. \quad \forall j = 1, \ldots, v. \tag{1.34}$$

However, given a particular design it is not always straightforward to check whether (1.34) holds. The following result of Baldi Antognini and Giovagnoli (2005) may be helpful:

Lemma 1.1 *Given a number $n_0 \geq 1$ of initial observations of each treatment, if*

$$\inf_{i>n_0} P\left(\delta_{j,i+1} = 1 \mid \delta^{(i)}, Y^{(i)}\right) > 0, \qquad \forall j = 1, \ldots, v,$$

then $\lim_{n\to\infty} N_{jn} = \infty \quad a.s.$ *for all* $j = 1, \ldots, v.$

As regards the asymptotic normality of the estimators, some "Central-Limit type" theorems have been proved for some of the adaptive designs proposed in the literature, for instance by Rosenberger and Sriram (1996). A general result holds, whose proof can be found in Baldi Antognini and Giovagnoli (2005):

Theorem 1.3 *When the responses belong to the regular exponential family (1.4) under Conditions 1, 2 and 3 of Section 1.3, if the allocation rule satisfies*

$$\lim_{n\to\infty} \frac{1}{n} \sum_{i=1}^{n} \Pr\left(\delta_{j,i+1} = 1 \mid \delta^{(i)}, Y^{(i)}\right) = t_j \quad a.s. \tag{1.35}$$

where $0 < t_j < 1$ *for all* $j = 1, \ldots, v$ *and the vector* $\mathbf{t} = (t_1, \ldots, t_v)^t$ *is non-random, as* $n \to \infty$ *the following is true:*

- $N_{jn} \to \infty \quad a.s. \quad$ *for all* $j = 1, \ldots, v$;
- $\boldsymbol{\pi}_n \to \mathbf{t} \quad a.s.$
- $\hat{\boldsymbol{\theta}}_n \to \boldsymbol{\theta} \quad a.s.$
- $\mathbf{M}(\boldsymbol{\theta} \mid \boldsymbol{\pi}_n) \to \boldsymbol{\Sigma}^{-1} = diag\left(\frac{t_1}{Var[Y_i|\delta_{i1}=1]}, \ldots, \frac{t_v}{Var[Y_i|\delta_{iv}=1]}\right) \quad a.s.$
- $\sqrt{n}(\hat{\boldsymbol{\theta}}_n - \boldsymbol{\theta}) \to^d N(\mathbf{0}; \boldsymbol{\Sigma})$.

Theorem 1.3 states that the possibility of asymptotic unconditional inference can be established by just looking at the design rule, namely checking whether (1.35) is true. Moreover, it gives the asymptotic properties of the estimators of the quantities of interest $\boldsymbol{\theta}$.

Theorem 1.3 is based on parametrization (1.17), and does not take into account the nuisance parameters, but sometimes it is necessary to estimate the nuisances as well; this point will find a further warrant in Chapter 3.

1.8.3 Asymptotic optimality of a sequential design

In order to simplify the notation, in this section we do not explicitly state the possible dependence of the targets on the unknown parameters.

Definition 1.2 *A sequential design for comparing v treatments will be said to be asymptotically optimal for conditional inference if*

$$\lim_{n\to\infty} \frac{\boldsymbol{N}_n}{n} = \boldsymbol{\pi}^* \quad a.s. \tag{1.36}$$

where $\boldsymbol{\pi}^*$ is a target treatment allocation that is optimal for conditional inference. Similarly, it will be denoted as asymptotically optimal for unconditional inference if

$$\lim_{n\to\infty} \frac{\boldsymbol{N}_n}{n} = \boldsymbol{\pi}^{**} \quad a.s. \tag{1.37}$$

where $\boldsymbol{\pi}^{**}$ is a target that is optimal for unconditional inference.

By continuity, under the assumptions of Theorem 1.3 the normalized conditional Fisher information matrix converges:

$$\lim_{n\to\infty} \mathbf{M}(\boldsymbol{\theta} \mid \boldsymbol{\pi}_n) \to \mathbf{M}(\boldsymbol{\theta} \mid \boldsymbol{t}^*) = \boldsymbol{\Sigma}^{-1} \quad a.s. \tag{1.38}$$

Thus, for a sequential design satisfying (1.35) the conditional and unconditional asymptotic variance of the ML estimators of $\boldsymbol{\theta}$ coincide and hence if a design is asymptotically optimal for conditional inference, it is also optimal unconditionally, and vice versa.

In some instances, as we shall see in the next chapters, it may be possible to show that the sequential design is asymptotically normal, i.e., there exist a target allocation $\boldsymbol{\pi}^0$ and a $(v \times v)$-dim symmetric matrix $\boldsymbol{\Lambda}$ such that

$$\sqrt{n}\left(\frac{\boldsymbol{N}_n}{n} - \boldsymbol{\pi}^0\right) \to^d N(\mathbf{0}; \boldsymbol{\Lambda}). \tag{1.39}$$

As anticipated at the end of Section 1.7, the asymptotic variance-covariance matrix $\boldsymbol{\Lambda}$ will in general affect the asymptotic inference. This will be explored in Chapter 3, with the definition of an *asymptotically best* design by Hu and Rosenberger (2006).

In any case, the asymptotic normality of a design is an indicator that the rate of convergence of the allocation proportion to the target $\boldsymbol{\pi}^0$ is $\sqrt{n}$, namely an indicator of slow convergence.

1.9 Some examples of convergence of designs

The following simple examples will help illustrate the asymptotic behaviour of some well-known and widely used sequential allocation rules when there are just two treatments A and B.

1.9.1 A likelihood-based design targeting Neyman's allocation

For the purpose of some of the examples in this Section we briefly sketch the Sequential Maximum Likelihood method, whose properties are studied at greater depth in Chapter 3.

Suppose that under treatments A and B, respectively, the responses are $Y_A \sim N(\mu_A; \sigma_A^2)$ and $Y_B \sim N(\mu_B; \sigma_B^2)$. The target that minimizes the variances of the estimator of the difference $\mu_A - \mu_B$ is Neyman's well-known allocation

$$\pi_N^* = \frac{\sigma_A}{\sigma_A + \sigma_B}.$$

Starting with an equal number n_0 of allocations of A and B, let $\hat{\sigma}_{Ai}$ and $\hat{\sigma}_{Bi}$ be the current MLEs of σ_A and σ_B at step $i \geq 2n_0$; at the next step, we assign the treatment A with probability equal to the estimated target:

$$\Pr\left(\delta_{i+1} = 1 \mid \delta^{(i)}, Y^{(i)}\right) = \frac{\hat{\sigma}_{Ai}}{\hat{\sigma}_{Ai} + \hat{\sigma}_{Bi}}.$$

In the rest of the book, this type of design will be called a Sequential Maximum Likelihood design. Since

$$\lim_{n\to\infty} \frac{1}{n} \sum_{i=1}^{n} \Pr\left(\delta_{i+1} = 1 \mid \delta^{(i)}, Y^{(i)}\right) = \frac{\sigma_A}{\sigma_A + \sigma_B} \quad a.s.$$

then by Theorem 1.3

$$\lim_{n\to\infty} \frac{N_{An}}{n} = \frac{\sigma_A}{\sigma_A + \sigma_B} \quad a.s.$$

so the design is asymptotically optimal.

Furthermore, let $\hat{\mu}_{An}$ and $\hat{\mu}_{Bn}$ denote the MLEs of μ_A and μ_B after n steps, then as $n \to \infty$

$$\sqrt{n}\begin{pmatrix} \hat{\mu}_{An} - \mu_A \\ \hat{\mu}_{Bn} - \mu_B \end{pmatrix} \to^d N\left(\begin{pmatrix} 0 \\ 0 \end{pmatrix}; \begin{pmatrix} \sigma_A^2\left(1 + \frac{\sigma_B}{\sigma_A}\right) & 0 \\ 0 & \sigma_B^2\left(1 + \frac{\sigma_A}{\sigma_B}\right) \end{pmatrix}\right)$$

and also

$$\sqrt{n}\left[(\hat{\mu}_{An} - \hat{\mu}_{Bn}) - (\mu_A - \mu_B)\right] \to^d N\left(0, (\sigma_A + \sigma_B)^2\right).$$

1.9.2 An asymptotically E-optimal design for the binary model

Suppose that the outcomes of the two treatments are binary with probabilities of success given by p_A and p_B. Assume we seek E-optimality, i.e., we want to minimize the maximum variance of the estimators of p_A and p_B, then the target proportion of allocations to A is

$$\pi_E^* = \frac{p_A q_A}{p_A q_A + p_B q_B}.$$

If we adopt the Sequential Maximum Likelihood design as in Section 1.9.1, namely assign at each step treatment A with probability given by the current MLE of the target

$$\Pr\left(\delta_{i+1}=1 \mid \delta^{(i)}, Z^{(i)}\right)=\frac{\hat{p}_{Ai}\,\hat{q}_{Ai}}{\hat{p}_{Ai}\,\hat{q}_{Ai}+\hat{p}_{Bi}\,\hat{q}_{Bi}}, \qquad \forall i \geq 2n_0,$$

then

$$\lim_{n\to\infty}\frac{N_{An}}{n}=\frac{p_Aq_A}{p_Aq_A+p_Bq_B} \quad a.s.$$

and therefore, as $n \to \infty$

$$\sqrt{n}\begin{pmatrix}\hat{p}_{An}-p_A\\ \hat{p}_{Bn}-p_B\end{pmatrix} \to^d N\left(\begin{pmatrix}0\\0\end{pmatrix};\begin{pmatrix}p_Aq_A\left(1+\frac{p_Bq_B}{p_Aq_A}\right) & 0\\ 0 & p_Bq_B\left(1+\frac{p_Aq_A}{p_Bq_B}\right)\end{pmatrix}\right).$$

1.10 The class of Markovian designs

We describe a type of adaptive design rules that obey a *Markov property* (Giovagnoli, 2004), namely either allocation-adaptive designs such that at each step the randomized allocation of the next treatment depends only on the most recent treatment allocation:

$$\Re\left(\boldsymbol{\delta}_{n+1} \mid \Im_n\right)=\Re(\boldsymbol{\delta}_{n+1} \mid \boldsymbol{\delta}_n), \qquad \forall n \geq 1 \tag{1.40}$$

or response-adaptive designs in which at each step randomization rule depends only on the most recent treatment allocation and relative outcome:

$$\Re(\boldsymbol{\delta}_{n+1} \mid \Im_n)=\Re(\boldsymbol{\delta}_{n+1} \mid \boldsymbol{\delta}_n, Y_n), \qquad \forall n \geq 1. \tag{1.41}$$

We now prove that combined with the conditional independence assumption (1.3), rule (1.41) guarantees that the sequence of design points of the experiment is a Markov chain. More precisely, the following holds true:

Lemma 1.2 *If (1.3) and (1.41) (or, alternatively, (1.40)) hold true, both the sequence $\{(\boldsymbol{\delta}_n, Y_n)\}_{n\in\mathbb{N}}$ and the sequence of the design points $\{\boldsymbol{\delta}_n\}_{n\in\mathbb{N}}$ are Markov chains.*

Proof *In this proof we only need to consider (1.41), since (1.40) can be regarded as a special case. From (1.3)*

$$\begin{aligned}\mathcal{L}(\boldsymbol{\delta}_{n+1}, Y_{n+1};\boldsymbol{\gamma}|\Im_n) &= \mathcal{L}(Y_{n+1};\boldsymbol{\gamma} \mid \boldsymbol{\delta}_{n+1}, \Im_n)\Re(\boldsymbol{\delta}_{n+1}|\Im_n)\\ &= \mathcal{L}(Y_{n+1};\boldsymbol{\gamma} \mid \boldsymbol{\delta}_{n+1})\Re(\boldsymbol{\delta}_{n+1}|\Im_n)\\ &= \mathcal{L}(Y_{n+1};\boldsymbol{\gamma} \mid \boldsymbol{\delta}_{n+1})\Re(\boldsymbol{\delta}_{n+1} \mid \boldsymbol{\delta}_n, Y_n)\\ &= \mathcal{L}(\boldsymbol{\delta}_{n+1}, Y_{n+1};\boldsymbol{\gamma} \mid \boldsymbol{\delta}_n, Y_n),\end{aligned}$$

which proves the first statement.

As to the Markov property for the sequence $\{\boldsymbol{\delta}_n\}_{n\in\mathbb{N}}$,

$$\Re\left(\boldsymbol{\delta}_{n+1} \mid \delta^{(n)}\right) = \int \mathcal{L}\left(\boldsymbol{\delta}_{n+1}, Y^{(n)} \mid \delta^{(n)}\right)$$

where the integration is with respect to the joint distribution of $Y^{(n)}$ *given* $\delta^{(n)}$. *Furthermore*

$$\begin{aligned}
\int \mathcal{L}\left(\boldsymbol{\delta}_{n+1}, Y^{(n)} \mid \delta^{(n)}\right) &= \int \Re\left(\boldsymbol{\delta}_{n+1} \mid Y^{(n)}, \delta^{(n)}\right) \mathcal{L}\left(Y^{(n)} \mid \delta^{(n)}\right) \\
&= \int \Re\left(\boldsymbol{\delta}_{n+1} \mid Y^{(n)}, \delta^{(n)}\right) \prod_{i=1}^{n} \mathcal{L}\left(Y_i \mid \boldsymbol{\delta}_i\right) \\
&= \int \Re\left(\boldsymbol{\delta}_{n+1} \mid Y_n, \boldsymbol{\delta}_n\right) \prod_{i=1}^{n} \mathcal{L}\left(Y_i \mid \boldsymbol{\delta}_i\right) \\
&= \int \mathcal{L}\left(\boldsymbol{\delta}_{n+1}, Y_n \mid \boldsymbol{\delta}_n\right) \prod_{i=1}^{n-1} \mathcal{L}\left(Y_i \mid \boldsymbol{\delta}_i\right) \\
&= \Re\left(\boldsymbol{\delta}_{n+1} \mid \boldsymbol{\delta}_n\right).
\end{aligned}$$

The definition of the Markov property can be generalized by replacing design *points* by design *statistics*. Assume that for a given design there is a sequence of generating design statistics $\left\{\boldsymbol{S}_n^d\right\}_{n\in\mathbb{N}}$ which satisfies the property

$$\Re\left(\boldsymbol{S}_{n+1}^d \mid \Im_n\right) = \Re\left(\boldsymbol{S}_{n+1}^d \mid \boldsymbol{S}_n^d, Y_n\right), \qquad n \geq 1, \tag{1.42}$$

where $\Re(\boldsymbol{S}_{n+1}^d \mid \Im_n)$ clearly denotes the probability distribution of $\boldsymbol{S}_{n+1}^d$ given the past history of the experiment. This property, together with the conditional independence of the outcomes (1.3), is sufficient to ensure that $\left\{\boldsymbol{S}_n^d\right\}_{n\in\mathbb{N}}$ is a Markov chain; the proof is identical to that of Lemma 1.2.

If the sequence $\{\boldsymbol{\delta}_n\}_{n\in\mathbb{N}}$ is an irreducible and positive recurrent, Markov chain, there will exist a stationary distribution $\boldsymbol{\xi}$. If the chain is also aperiodic, by the Law of Large Numbers for Markov chains the experiment will converge to $\boldsymbol{\xi}$. In other words, the randomization procedure will tend to a target treatment allocation, which can be described as the *asymptotic design*. Furthermore, further conditions ensure that often a Central Limit Theorem holds for the design (Hoel et al., 1972).

1.11 Some examples of Markovian designs

The following examples refer to designs for which either (1.41) or (1.42) holds. They illustrate the theoretical properties discussed in Sections 1.5 and 1.8. We stress that the Markovian designs briefly sketched here are introduced only as examples; their properties are studied at greater depth in Chapters 2 and 3.

1.11.1 Efron's coin

Consider two treatments A and B with mean responses μ_A and μ_B and equal variance σ^2. As already pointed out, balancing the treatments is often an optimal target; this target does not depend on the unknown parameters. Efron (1971) has proposed his by now widely known *Biased Coin* design (BCD), namely a sequential randomized design for comparing two treatments that offers a trade-off between imbalance and randomness.

Let $D_n = \sum_{i=1}^n \delta_i = N_{An} - N_{Bn}$ be the difference in assignments between the two treatment arms after n assignments. The sequence $\{D_n\}_{n\in\mathbb{N}}$ is a generating design statistic for the experiment. At each step Efron's BCD randomizes the next assignment by means of the hypothetical tossing of a biased coin with probability $p \geqslant 1/2$ which favours the treatment so far under-represented. Formally

$$\Pr\left(\delta_{n+1} = 1 \mid \delta^{(n)}\right) = \begin{cases} p, & D_n < 0, \\ 1/2, & D_n = 0, \\ 1-p, & D_n > 0. \end{cases} \tag{1.43}$$

This design is allocation-adaptive, and $\{D_n\}_{n\in\mathbb{N}}$ satisfies the Markov property (1.42) since $D_{n+1} = D_n \pm 1$ so that $\Re\left(D_{n+1} \mid \delta_1 \ldots, \delta_n\right) = \Re\left(D_{n+1} \mid D_n\right)$. Hence $\{D_n\}_{n\in\mathbb{N}}$ is a Markov chain.

The asymptotic behaviour of the BCD is provided by the steady-state properties of $\{D_n\}_{n\in\mathbb{N}}$, in particular it can be shown that $n^{-1}D_n \to 0$ almost surely as n tends to infinity, i.e., the BCD converges to balance almost surely. As regards parametric inference, the analysis of data obtained by this experiment can be conditioned on the observed numbers of allocations to the two treatments. If, after n steps, we have observed n_A and n_B assignments to the two treatments, then the variances of the estimators

$$\hat{\mu}_{An} = \frac{\sum_{i=1}^n \delta_i Y_i}{n_A} \quad \text{and} \quad \hat{\mu}_{Bn} = \frac{\sum_{i=1}^n (1-\delta_i) Y_i}{n_B}$$

are the usual ones, namely σ^2/n_A and σ^2/n_B, respectively.

Because of the random nature of the design, randomization-based inference is also possible, and Markaryan and Rosenberger (2010) have obtained exact finite sample results for this design, but this type of inference is not discussed in this book.

1.11.2 Zelen's play-the-winner

For binary responses, one of the most popular designs is the so-called Play-the-Winner (PW) rule (Zelen, 1969), with its roots in *bandit* problems (see Rosenberger and Lachin (2002)): a success on a given treatment leads to assigning the same treatment to the next statistical unit, while a failure means switching to the other treatment, whereas the first allocation is determined by tossing a fair coin. Given the most recent allocation and outcome, at each step the choice of the next assignment is deterministic and is given by

$$\Pr\left(\delta_{n+1} = 1 \mid \delta^{(n)}, Y^{(n)}\right) = \Pr\left(\delta_{n+1} = 1 \mid \delta_n, Y_n\right), \quad n \geq 1. \tag{1.44}$$

It is easy to see that the sequence of probabilities $\{\Pr(\delta_{n+1}=1 \mid \delta_n, Y_n)\}_{n\in\mathbb{N}}$ is a homogeneous Markov chain on the state space $\{0;1\}$ with transition matrix

$$P=\begin{pmatrix} p_B & q_B \\ q_A & p_A \end{pmatrix}.$$

It is straightforward to check that the stationary law is Bernoulli $Be\left(q_B/(q_A+q_B)\right)$, so that from the ergodic theorem for Markov chains

$$\lim_{n\to\infty}\frac{1}{n}\sum_{i=1}^{n}\Pr(\delta_{i+1}=1 \mid \delta_i, Y_i)=\frac{q_B}{q_A+q_B} \quad a.s. \tag{1.45}$$

and hence condition (1.35) holds true. Then, by Theorem 1.3

$$\lim_{n\to\infty}\frac{N_{An}}{n}=\frac{q_B}{q_A+q_B} \quad a.s.$$

The quantity $q_B/(q_A+q_B)$ is commonly referred to as the relative risk of B, and similarly for A. The outstanding feature of the PW design is that the treatment allocation of A converges to the relative risk of B, and conversely, which implies that in the long run a majority of units will receive the better treatment and makes the PW rule an appealing one. We shall deal with this design and its modifications in more detail in Chapter 4.

The asymptotic distribution of the ML estimators is given by

$$\begin{pmatrix} \sqrt{n}[\hat{p}_{An}-p_A] \\ \sqrt{n}[\hat{p}_{Bn}-p_B] \end{pmatrix} \to^d N\left(\begin{bmatrix} 0 \\ 0 \end{bmatrix}; \begin{bmatrix} p_Aq_A(1+\frac{q_A}{q_B}) & 0 \\ 0 & p_Bq_B(1+\frac{q_B}{q_A}) \end{bmatrix}\right).$$

It is useful to stress the different behaviours of the asymptotic variance of estimators in the allocation-adaptive and response-adaptive cases. In the former (see Section 1.11.1) there is no difference with non-sequential designs, whereas for the response-adaptive case of this section and of Section 1.9.1, the asymptotic variance of each treatment estimator does not depend just on the variance of the responses to that treatment, but also on the variability induced by the design; in particular, there is an extra variability component related to the variance of the responses to the other treatment.

1.11.3 An "up-and-down" design

The Up-and-Down designs are examples of randomization rules that depend on the observed data, but are different from the ones considered so far in that the v treatments are ordered. They will be studied in depth in Chapter 3: here we mention just a simple case to illustrate the Markov property.

Assume the probability of a positive response in a binary experiment to be a strictly increasing function $Q(x)$ of a stimulus x, for instance the level of a potentially lethal or teratogenous drug. The *quantal response curve* $y=Q(x)$ is unknown and a typical statistical problem is the search for a given "quantile" of Q, namely $x_{(\Gamma)} =$

$Q^{-1}(\Gamma)$, where $Q^{-1}(p) = \inf\{x : Q(x) \geq p,\}, 0 < p < 1$. Let $D = \{d_0, \ldots, d_M\}$ denote the set of available treatment levels, in increasing order, and assume $Q(d_0) = 0$, $Q(d_M) = 1$ and $0 < Q(d_k) < 1$ for all $0 < k < M$. By a slight change of notation, let X_n denote the treatment level applied at step n and let Y_n be the corresponding observation, taking values 0 or 1. The following decision rule is the one given by Durham and Flournoy (1994):

Rule DF: choose a starting point X_1 in D, at each step $n \geq 1$

- conditionally on $X_n = d_k$ $(k = 0, 1, \ldots, M-1)$ and $Y_n = 0$

$$\begin{aligned} X_{n+1} &= d_{k+1} \quad \text{with probability } \alpha = \min\left\{\frac{\Gamma}{1-\Gamma}, 1\right\} \ (0 < \alpha \leq 1), \\ X_{n+1} &= d_k \quad \text{with probability } 1 - \alpha; \end{aligned}$$

- conditionally on $X_n = d_k$ $(k = 1, \ldots, M)$ and $Y_n = 1$

$$\begin{aligned} X_{n+1} &= d_{k-1} \text{ with probability } \beta = \min\left\{\frac{1-\Gamma}{\Gamma}, 1\right\} \quad (0 < \beta \leq 1), \\ X_{n+1} &= d_k \quad \text{with probability } 1 - \beta. \end{aligned}$$

Rule DF satisfies the Markov property (1.41) hence the sequence $\{X_n\}_{n \in \mathbb{N}}$ of allocated treatments created by this rule is a Markov chain – more precisely, it is a random walk – on the state space D, with transition probabilities

$$\begin{aligned} p_k &= \Pr(X_{n+1} = d_{k+1} \mid X_n = d_k) = \alpha(1 - Q_k) \\ q_k &= \Pr(X_{n+1} = d_{k-1} \mid X_n = d_k) = \beta Q_k \\ r_k &= \Pr(X_{n+1} = d_k \mid X_n = d_k) = 1 - p_k - q_k, \end{aligned}$$

for $k = 2, \ldots M-1$. Unless $\alpha = \beta = 1$, the Markov chain $\{X_n\}_{n \in \mathbb{N}}$ can be shown to have a stationary distribution $\boldsymbol{\xi} = \{\xi_k = \xi(d_k) : k = 0, \ldots, M\}$ given by the equilibrium equations

$$\begin{aligned} \xi_k &= \xi_{k-1}\left(\frac{p_{k-1}}{q_k}\right) \qquad k = 1, \ldots, M, \qquad (1.46) \\ \xi_0 &= \left[1 + \sum_{i=1}^{M} \prod_{k=1}^{i} \frac{p_{k-1}}{q_k}\right]^{-1}. \end{aligned}$$

Denoting by $N_n(d_k)$ the number of assignments of treatment level d_k up to step n, by the Law of Large Numbers for Markov chains

$$\lim_{n \to \infty} \frac{N_n(d_k)}{n} \to \xi_k \qquad a.s. \qquad \forall k = 0, 1, \ldots, M.$$

So, the asymptotic behaviour of the treatment allocations is described by $\boldsymbol{\xi}$. Besides, by the Central Limit Theorem for Markov chains as $n \to \infty$

$$\sqrt{n}\left(\frac{N_n(d_k)}{n} - \xi_k\right) \to^d N(0, v_k), \qquad \forall k = 0, 1, \ldots, M. \qquad (1.47)$$

In addition, the mode d_m of the stationary distribution is such that

$$d_{m-1} < x_{(\Gamma)} \leq d_{m+1}. \tag{1.48}$$

Inequalities (1.48) imply that the mode d_m of $\boldsymbol{\xi}$ can be used as an approximation of $x_{(\Gamma)}$.

1.12 Sequential designs and stopping rules

In all the previous sections we have discussed sequential designs with a predetermined value of n. This is a common feature of most practical implementations, since it is useful to know the sample size in advance for administrative reasons. The introduction of a rule for stopping is often more efficient, since it may lead to fewer observations and savings in terms of budget and/or human effort, but obviously makes the sample size random. Stopping rules play a central role in the theory of sequential analysis (see Siegmund (1985)), which goes back to Wald's contributions (Wald, 1947) in the context of statistical quality control for industrial inspection.

A simple example of stopping rule is the classical "inverse sampling"(see Smith (1982)), namely the experiment goes on until a given random event is observed. This is implemented in numerous branches of statistics: sampling plans (Haldane, 1945; Hawkins, 2001), clinical trials (Wei, 1978b; Bandyopadhyay and Biswas, 1997a,b, 2000, 2003), selection procedures (Sobel and Weiss, 1971; Berry and Sobel, 1973), etc. A particular case is the so-called *binomial inverse sampling*. Under this scheme the experiment stops as soon as a fixed number s of successes is observed. An inverse sampling scheme is also introduced by Tweedie (1957) for normal responses: he proposes to stop the experiment when the sum of the observations reaches a given threshold.

In our context of comparative experiments with $v \geq 2$ populations (the treatment arms), the design consists in defining both the sequential allocation rule and the rule for stopping the experiment. The definition of adaptive design needs to be extended if we wish to include stopping too. Let $\mathbb{1}_{\{\mathcal{A}_k\}}$ be the indicator function of the event $\mathcal{A}_k$ ="stopping the experiment after assigning a treatment at step k and observing the data". The design will be described by $\Pr(\delta_{j1} = 1)$ for $j = 1, \ldots, v$ and the sequences of probabilities:

$$\left\{\Pr\left(\delta_{j,i+1} = 1 \mid \boldsymbol{\delta}^{(i)}, \boldsymbol{Y}^{(i)}, \mathbb{1}_{\{\mathcal{A}_i\}} = 0\right), j = 1, \ldots, v\right\}_{i \geq 1}$$

and

$$\left\{\Pr\left(\mathbb{1}_{\{\mathcal{A}_i\}} = 1 \mid \boldsymbol{\delta}^{(i)}, \boldsymbol{Y}^{(i)}\right)\right\}_{i \geq 1}.$$

Ideally, the same distinction between *allocation-adaptive* and *response-adaptive*, discussed at the end of Section 1.2 for allocation rules, could be made for stopping rules, namely the stopping rule could depend on just the past allocations, for instance stopping when each treatment has been assigned at least a given number of times, but in practice the only rules that are used are the ones that take into account the observed data.

Here are a few examples of combinations of an adaptive allocation rule and a stopping rule.

Example 1.2 (Sobel and Weiss (1971)) *In a binary response trial for comparing two treatments, the PW allocation rule can be combined with an inverse sampling scheme, stopping the experiment when a fixed number of successes are observed from either of the two treatments. The expected total number of observations can be calculated.*

Example 1.3 (Hoel (1972)) *Sobel and Weiss's procedure can be modified as follows: the PW allocation rule is combined with a stopping rule, which takes the numbers of both successes and failures into account, stopping the experiment when the number of successes of a treatment added to the failures of the other exceeds a fixed threshold. This design has good general properties: in particular, excessive sample sizes are avoided when the success probabilities are small.*

These procedures have been further modified by various authors, e.g. Fushimi (1973), Berry and Sobel (1973), Kiefer and Weiss (1974) and Nordbrock (1976), who have analyzed the PW allocation in conjunction with more complex stopping rules.

Example 1.4 (Wei and Durham (1978)) *The allocation rule is Randomized Play-the-Winner (RPW) (to be introduced in Chapter 4) and the stopping rule is the one of Example 1.3.*

Example 1.5 (Bandyopadhyay and Biswas (1997a,b, 2000, 2002, 2003)) *In a series of papers, Bandyopadhyay and Biswas suggest that to test for the equality of the effects of two treatments in binary response trials, one could use the RPW allocation (Wei, 1978a) and the stopping rule proposed by Sobel and Weiss (1971).*

Example 1.6 (Baldi Antognini and Giovagnoli (2005)) *The following stopping rule is suggested for comparative experiments with responses belonging to the exponential family: stop when the absolute value of the sum of the responses relative to each treatment T_j reaches a given value $r_j \in \mathbb{R}^+$*

$$N = \inf\left\{ n \in \mathbb{N},\ s.t. \left| \sum_{i=1}^{n} \delta_{ji} Y_i \right| \geq r_j, \quad (j = 1, \ldots, v) \right\}. \tag{1.49}$$

For a binary response trial, rule (1.49) leads to setting a lower threshold for the number of observed successes of each treatment, which in the case of just one treatment would be the classical binomial inverse sampling. For normal responses, rule (1.49) corresponds to the inverse sampling scheme proposed by Tweedie (1957). Combining the Sequential Maximum Likelihood design (see Chapter 3) with this stopping rule, the authors show that the strong consistency and asymptotical normality of the MLEs still hold approximately.

Stopping at predetermined time periods and carrying out an *interim analysis* of the data gathered so far to decide whether to continue or not is often done in clinical trials, especially when monitoring for futility or adverse events. When testing for treatment equality, more complex decision rules have been devised that allow the scientist, at each stage, to either stop, accepting or rejecting the null hypothesis, or continue the experiment (triangular test). These rules consist in setting boundaries for a predetermined test statistic so that some error probability requirements are satisfied. There is a rich literature on this topic, starting from Pocock (1977), O'Brien and Fleming (1979), Whitehead (1997) and Jennison and Turnbull (2000). These designs, known as *group-sequential designs*, in general do not consider treatment allocations other than equal size randomization. For normal data with known variances, however, Jennison and Turnbull (2001) showed that response-adaptive randomization can be incorporated into a general family of group sequential tests without affecting the error probabilities. Zhu and Hu (2010) study both theoretical properties and finite sample properties of some designs which combine sequential monitoring with response-adaptive randomization.

Recently the attention has focussed on stochastic curtailment (stopping the experiment when a particular decision is highly likely given the current data) and in particular on rules based on conditional power when stopping for futility (Lachin, 2005) in bio-pharmaceutical experiments. In this book we shall not deal with this topic any further.

1.13 Some practical issues in the implementation of adaptive designs

Adaptive designs are used in actual practice, especially in clinical and pharmaceutical contexts: a renowned case is the Michigan ECMO trial (Bartlett et al., 1985). Researchers working for pharmaceutical companies tend to express enthusiastic support of adaptive designs, but there have been several criticisms too. Korn and Freidlin (2011) address response-adaptive randomization in a two-armed trial in which the randomization ratio changes during a period of time on the basis of the current Bayesian probability that an arm is the better treatment. They use simulations to investigate whether this adaptive approach is better than the fixed randomization approach and conclude that the adaptive approach is not superior. Berry (2011), however, disproves their conclusion.

In any case, suitable implementation of the adaptive design methodology requires particular attention, even more so when the design rule is based on the observed outcomes (i.e., for response-adaptive designs and the CARA procedures of Chapter 6). For a start, adaptive designs are more susceptible to population drifts during a period of time, as pointed out by many authors. Also, delayed responses often occur in a real context. From a mathematical viewpoint there are no difficulties in incorporating a delay mechanism for the responses into the design adaptation (Hu and Rosenberger, 2006). Indeed, in this case every update of the design (in terms of sequential estimation of the unknown model parameters and/or urn reinforcement, which we introduce in Chapter 2) will be made only when the responses become available. Thus, the crucial question concerns the amount of collected information during the recruitment period. Several authors have explored the effects of delayed responses on both i) the design variability and ii) the statistical efficiency of the usual inferential procedures (see for instance Bai et al. (2002a), Zhang and Rosenberger (2006), Zhang et al. (2007a) and Hu et al. (2008)). Roughly speaking, all the asymptotic properties of such designs still hold provided that the delay mechanism of the outcomes is not dominant with respect to the subjects entry mechanism, i.e., the incoming information cannot be undermined by the delayed responses. For instance, in a clinical trial if we assume that the subjects entries are iid and follow a uniform distribution in a given time interval, it is sufficient to assume that the delay process has at least an exponential decay in order to ensure that the decay cannot be too large with respect to the enrollment. These results hold asymptotically; however, for small samples delayed responses might have a substantial impact. Indeed, as shown by Zhang and Rosenberger (2006), the variance of the treatment allocation proportions increases as the average delay grows, but it has a negligible effect in terms of the power when testing for equality, provided that, during the trial, at least 60% of the responses of the allocated units are available.

As regards another practical issue, missing data are perhaps less likely to occur in a sequential experiment which in general is monitored very closely, but the existence of this problem must be acknowledged. There are many popular statistical techniques to handle missing values in the literature which have been proposed and analyzed in the context of fixed sample designs (see for instance Little and Rubin (2002) and Molenberghs and Kenward (2007)). Understanding the reasons why data are missing helps in analyzing the remaining data. If values are missing at random, the data sample may still be representative of the population, but if the values are missing systematically, the analysis is harder. To our knowledge, a clear investigation of the effect of missing data on response-adaptive procedures as well as on the corresponding inference is still an open problem to this date.

1.14 Simulating adaptive designs

We would like to end this chapter with some personal comments on computer experiments.

Simulating physical experiments by means of a computer program for the purpose of acquiring information that is either impossible, or too long, or too expensive to obtain from a real-life experiment has become a more and more widespread activity since computers have come into common use. Thanks also to the advent of new powerful software, this type of simulation is taking place and indeed is recommended in clinical trials too (Kimko and Duffull, 2003; Taylor and Bosch, 1990; Holford et al., 2010); for an introduction see Krause (2010). In the context of this book, however, we wish to focus on a different type of simulation studies, whose purpose is to evaluate the performance of one or more particular adaptive designs, possibly with a mind to choosing one of them before performing the experiment. Simulation-based approaches are also resorted to in order to study the power of a test or the behaviour of some estimators, especially in finite samples.

In principle, computer simulation is a formidable tool to investigate the properties of adaptive designs. Simulation studies are meta-experiments, namely experiments (done on the computer) to observe the stochastic behaviour of a designed experiment. The simulation usually consists in running the computer experiment according to the chosen design, mimicking the random behaviour of "nature" by means of the statistical model, after choosing some suitable values of the parameters as the "true" values, and also mimicking the randomization mechanism, if present in the design.

Some computer experiments are of a confirmatory nature: they are performed to show that a given experimental design behaves as predicted by the theory. They serve an illustrative and didactic purpose. However, most simulations are genuinely exploratory: they are intended to investigate some unknown features of the design. By repeating the computer experiment a large number N of times, the stochastic distribution of the design is observed empirically and the performance characteristics of interest, which are in general means or variances of chosen indicators or the frequency behaviour of the test statistic, and thus are functions of this empirical distribution, are calculated numerically. Well known foundational controversies pertaining to the meaning of *repeated experiments* lose their *raison d'être* in this set-up, and the frequentist philosophy gains a new momentum. More specifically, simulations are usually carried out in the adaptive design context in order to

a) investigate some convergence properties, e.g., see whether in the long run the design approaches a predefined target, and how fast;

b) compare two or more different designs with respect to some measure of their performance. This may refer to the asymptotic behaviour or, more frequently, to the small sample one, which is more difficult to establish on a theoretical basis.

Since a simulation study is a meta-experiment, one would expect the statistical design community to have devoted more attention to the design of simulation projects. So far, however, this research area is still in its early days, and statisticians do not seem to have capitalized on statistical design ideas for making their simulations as effective and informative as possible. Statements of the type: "Our simulations show..." without any further details are not unusual, while a scientific report stating "An experiment of ours shows... ", with no description of the real-life experiment itself, would be unacceptable.

The particular issue of choosing the "true" values of the unknown parameters may prove really crucial. In simulating allocation-adaptive designs, we do not always have to choose parameters values, as some measures of performance like lack of balance, loss, and selection bias depend on the design alone, not on the responses. However, even for allocation-adaptive designs, in order to assess inferential features like the power and the variances of the estimators we need to simulate the behaviour of the responses too. This is always the case when the designs are response-adaptive. Three common ways of choosing the values of the unknown parameters are

a) best guesses;

b) estimates from real data available in the literature, especially when the design in question is a "re-design" of a well-known real life experiment (see e.g. Atkinson and Biswas (2014));

c) values that form a grid covering the whole parameter space.

Method b), although more sensible than a), may lead to wrong conclusions, as we shall discuss in Section 4.2.3 about the RPW rule with two treatments; indeed, the asymptotic properties of the RPW design in terms of both the rate of convergence and the asymptotic distribution depend on the values of the treatment effects, and therefore it would be reckless to draw conclusions from simulations based on method b). Method c) seems safer, although as we know from the theory of physical experimental designs, it may be far from ideal.

Apart from the possibility of being misleading, the main problem with adaptive design simulations is that they are often inconclusive, as one can apperceive in the book by Atkinson and Biswas (2014), where comparisons via simulations play a major part.

2

Randomization procedures that are functions of the past allocations

2.1 Introduction

This chapter is about adaptive allocation rules which depend on the past history of the experiment only through the sequence of previous treatment assignments. They have the advantage that the whole experiment can be designed in advance, before collecting the responses, and inference may be conditional on the design. Sequential procedures where the choice of the next design point is made on the basis of the previous points are, for instance, the Wynn–Fedorov designs for the linear model (Wynn, 1972; Fedorov, 1972), which at each step add design points where the variance of the predicted response is highest so as to converge to D-optimality. For instance in the case of a homoscedastic linear model for estimating v treatments, at each step the Wynn–Fedorov algorithm would choose to observe the under-represented treatment, with no preference in case of a tie. However, the Wynn–Fedorov designs are deterministic, whereas in this book we are concerned with randomized assignments.

Another important issue is balance: in a large number of comparative experiments the researchers would like to achieve a balanced or near balanced allocation among the treatments. Balance is often related to inferential optimality (see Appendix A). However, it is fairly intuitive that balance and randomness are conflicting demands, as we show in Section 2.2.

The main topic of the present Chapter is allocation-adaptive designs intended to achieve some balance and maintain a good degree of randomness in the assignments. It is not surprising that these designs have been studied mainly in the context of randomized clinical trials (see for instance Berger et al. (2003) and Sverdlov and Rosenberger (2013b)). The requirement of a suitable trade-off between inferential optimality and unpredictability is particularly cogent for Phase III trials, where patients are enrolled sequentially and the total sample size is often a priori unknown, so that keeping a reasonable degree of balance at each step, while maintaining a good degree of overall randomness, could be crucial to allow the experiment to be stopped at any time in a good inferential setting. The *Handbook of Adaptive Designs in Pharmaceutical and Clinical Development* devotes a chapter (Biswas and Bhattacharya, 2011) to such allocation rules.

In order to compare different designs, the need has arisen to find ways of measuring the degree of randomness and the degree of imbalance of an allocation rule.

Section 2.3 deals with indicators of imbalance and predictability suggested in the literature.

Fundamental randomization devices that guarantee a suitable amount of randomness in the treatment allocation process while driving the assignments towards balance are the ones that have stemmed from the pioneering work of Efron (1971) and Wei (1978b), namely the biased coin designs on the one hand and the urn designs on the other (see Atkinson (1982), Chen (1999, 2000), Smith (1984a,b), Soares and Wu (1983), Wei (1978a)). Both names – *biased coin* and *urn* designs – originate from traditional ways of describing the allocation mechanisms. Efron's Biased Coin (BCD), already mentioned in Chapter 1, and its developments were born for comparing just two treatments: at each step the treatments are assigned according to the toss of a biased coin that favours the under-represented one with a probability linked to the current imbalance. In the urn designs, at every step the treatment allocation is randomized by selecting a ball at random from an urn containing a given number of balls of several types, one for each available treatment: when a ball of a given type is drawn, the corresponding treatment gets assigned. The evolution of the urn is governed by the so-called *addition rule*, which specifies i) whether the chosen ball will be replaced in the urn or not and ii) how many balls of each type will be added, if any, to the urn. The initial urn composition together with the addition rule are the crucial ingredients which determine the evolution of the urn process and of the design itself. Clearly, nowadays these randomization methods are no longer implemented by physical urns or coins, but rather by a computer programme. Thus there is no longer the restriction, say, of adding (or subtracting) an integer number of balls.

Section 2.4 of this chapter is about biased coin designs. They fall into two large classes: the Adaptive BCD suggested by Wei (1978a) and the Adjustable BCD proposed by Baldi Antognini and Giovagnoli (2004). Section 2.5 deals with urn designs which are allocation-adaptive, such as the Generalized Friedman's Urn (GFU), sometimes referred to as the Generalized Pólya Urn, the Ehrenfest Design (ED) and some of their extensions. In this chapter we restrict the presentation to designs with just $v = 2$ treatments, but in several cases the definitions and results can be extended to more than two. A much more thorough account of urn designs is given in Hu and Rosenberger (2006); in this chapter we only present the main ideas: the topic will be further developed in the next chapters of the book in the context of response-adaptive designs.

2.2 Randomization and balance as conflicting demands

From a statistical perspective, a fundamental aim of a design is to optimize inference about the treatments. As mentioned in Appendix A, if the inferential goal is estimation of the treatment effects, under the linear model assumptions the balanced design is *universally optimal*, i.e., it minimizes all convex optimality criteria. Balancing the allocations of the treatment arms is also optimal under several criteria related to testing. Balance is also desirable for more general statistical models. In fact, it is always D-optimal for responses belonging to the exponential family (see Remark 1.1in Chapter 1). Moreover, a balanced design may be close to being A-optimal even for binary responses (see Section 1.7 in Chapter 1).

Let there be two treatments A and B and suppose we have chosen a sequential randomization rule $\Pr(\delta_{n+1} = 1 \mid \delta_1 \ldots, \delta_n)$. Consider the stochastic process $\{D_n\}_{n\in\mathbb{N}}$, where $D_n = N_{An} - N_{Bn}$, whose probabilistic structure and properties will depend on the adopted allocation rule. As mentioned in Section 1.11.1, the sequence $\{D_n\}_{n\in\mathbb{N}}$ is easily seen to be a generating statistic sequence for the design and for all $n \in \mathbb{N}$

$$\Pr(D_n = k) > 0 \quad \text{iff} \quad |k| \leq n \ \text{ where } n \text{ and } k \text{ have the same parity.}$$

Ideally, the behaviour of $\{D_n\}_{n\in\mathbb{N}}$ should be close to 0 at each step, in order to guarantee near-balance for any sample size, but if the drive towards balance is stronger, then the random component in the allocations will be smaller, and vice versa. In order to construct a sequential design which is perfectly balanced at each step, the treatment allocations need to be partially or completely deterministic. For instance, the design that assigns treatment A at each odd number of steps and B in the remaining cases, namely

$$\delta_n = \begin{cases} 1 & n = 2k-1 \\ 0 & n = 2k \end{cases} \tag{2.1}$$

generates the following sequence of assignments $(AB)(AB)(AB)(AB)\ldots$ Obviously this procedure is perfectly balanced at each stage, since $|D_n| = 0$ or $|D_n| = 1$ if n is even or odd, respectively, but the entire sequence of assignments is deterministic and so completely predictable. A design which gets often recommended is the Permuted Block Design of size 2 (PBD_2): every odd allocation is randomized with probability 1/2 to either treatment, while the next assignment is made deterministically to the under-represented treatment, so that balance is guaranteed for each pair of subjects. Under this choice $\delta_1, \delta_3, \delta_5, \ldots$ are iid Bernoulli random variables $Be(1/2)$ and $\delta_2 = 1 - \delta_1, \delta_4 = 1 - \delta_3, \delta_6 = 1 - \delta_5, \ldots$, which generates sequences of assignments of the type $(AB)(BA)(AB)(AB)\ldots$. Thus at each step PBD_2 is perfectly balanced, i.e., $|D_n| \leq 1$ for every n, but now only 50% of the assignments are deterministic. Clearly, the size of the blocks could be chosen to be greater than 2, by considering a randomization sequence of 4, 8 or 10 units; but for any chosen block size s, PBD_s ensures balance only when the sample size is a multiple of s, not otherwise, and the deterministic component in the allocation process could be very relevant (see for instance Efron (1971), Rosenberger and Lachin (2002), Bailey and Nelson (2003), Salama et al. (2008), Zhao and Weng (2011b)).

On the other side, the completely randomized design CR assigns either treatment to each statistical unit with probability 1/2, independently of the previous allocations. Under CR, $\{\delta_n\}_{n\geq 1}$ is a sequence of iid Bernoulli random variables $Be(1/2)$ so that, from the Strong Law of Large Numbers

$$\lim_{n\to\infty} n^{-1} D_n = 0 \quad a.s.$$

CR may be seen as an ideal trade-off between optimality and randomness, since the design is completely unpredictable at each step and the relative imbalance vanishes asymptotically. However, from the Central Limit Theorem for iid random variables, as n tends to infinity

$$n^{-1/2} D_n \to^d Z \,,$$

where Z is a standard normal variable. Therefore the rate of convergence towards balance is slow and for small samples CR may generate large departures from balance which may induce a substantial loss of precision (Cumberland and Royall, 1988). Again, this shows the clash between randomization and balance.

For both CR and PBD_2, the Markov condition (1.42) is satisfied by process $\{D_n\}_{n\in\mathbb{N}}$. More specifically,

- under design PBD_2, $\{D_n\}_{n\in\mathbb{N}}$ takes values in $\{-1;0;1\}$ and is a symmetric random walk with completely reflecting barriers at 1 and -1; the stationary distribution puts probability 0.25, 0.5 and 0.25, respectively, at the support points;
- under the CR design, $\{D_n\}_{n\in\mathbb{N}}$ is a symmetric random walk on the integers; the support of D_n diverges as n increases and there does not exist a stationary distribution.

Most of the designs that we present in this chapter will also be Markovian and lie between these two "extreme" cases, namely $\text{PBD}_2$and CR.

2.3 Indicators of balance and randomness

In order to compare different sequential designs with respect to their degrees of balance and randomization, several measures of imbalance and of lack of randomness have been introduced (see for instance Burman (1996), Chen (1999), Zhao and Weng (2011a), Zhao et al. (2012)). Some refer to the behaviour of the design at step n, for each n, others take into account the average behaviour in the first n steps. Because the design is random, so are the measures involved and a common approach is to use their expectations as the indicators of interest. The comparison of designs usually takes place by means of a graphical display of the respective values of the indicators as n varies, as in Atkinson (2014).

2.3.1 Measures of imbalance

The treatment imbalance of a sequential design at step n is $|D_n|$, and all the measures of the degree of imbalance are some transformation of the random quantity $|D_n|$. The imbalance performance of a design is evaluated by considering the expected value of such transformation with respect to its distribution. For a start, natural indicators of imbalance at step n are $E[|D_n|]$ and $E[D_n^2]$. Other instances are (Zhao et al., 2012):

a) the probability of achieving exact balance at step $n > 1$, $\Pr(|D_n = 0|)$,

b) the standard deviation of the imbalance $|D_n|$ at the end of the trial,

c) the maximum absolute imbalance in the entire sequence, $\max_{\{1\le i\le n\}} |D_i|$.

If the allocation rule treats A and B symmetrically, then

$$\Pr(D_n = k) = \Pr(D_n = -k), \qquad \text{for all } k \in \mathbb{Z}$$

and thus

$$E[D_n] = 0, \qquad \text{for all } n \in \mathbb{N} \tag{2.2}$$

so that $Var[D_n] = E[D_n^2]$ and the standard deviation of the treatment imbalance at step n is $\sqrt{E[D_n^2]}$.

Measures of *average imbalance* are $n^{-1}\sum_{i=1}^{n} E[|D_i|]$ (see Chen (1999)) and

$$\frac{1}{n}\sum_{i=1}^{n} E[D_i^2] = \frac{1}{n}\sum_{i=1}^{n} Var[D_i].$$

Example 2.1 *For deterministic designs like $ABABA\ldots$ and PDB$_2$ the imbalance is*

$$E[|D_n|] = Var[D_n] = \begin{cases} 0, & n \text{ even} \\ 1, & n \text{ odd} \end{cases},$$

so that the average imbalance is

$$\frac{1}{n}\sum_{i=1}^{n} E[|D_i|] = \frac{1}{n}\sum_{i=1}^{n} Var[D_n] = \begin{cases} \frac{1}{2}, & n \text{ even} \\ \frac{1}{2} + \frac{1}{2n}, & n \text{ odd} \end{cases}.$$

Thus, both procedures are perfectly balanced.

For the completely randomized design

$$Var[D_n] = n \qquad \text{and} \qquad \frac{1}{n}\sum_{i=1}^{n} Var[D_i] = \frac{n+1}{2},$$

which clearly diverge asymptotically. The indicators $E[|D_n|]$ and $n^{-1}\sum_{i=1}^{n} E[|D_i|]$ can be derived with tedious calculations and similarly shown to diverge.

There are other indicators of imbalance which take into account the sample size explicitly. For instance, under a linear homoscedastic model for the responses, balance is optimal, so that optimality criteria, which are measures of the lack of inferential precision, and their expectations, can also be regarded as indirect imbalance measures (after a suitable standardization, if necessary).

Example 2.2 *Adopting the linear homoscedastic model*

$$E[Y_i] = \delta_i \mu_A + (1-\delta_i)\mu_B\,, \qquad Var[Y_i] = \sigma^2 \qquad i \ge 1, \tag{2.3}$$

after n assignments the conditional variance-covariance matrix of the OLS parameter estimators $\hat{\mu}_{An}$ and $\hat{\mu}_{Bn}$ is

$$\mathbf{V}(\hat{\mu}_A, \hat{\mu}_B) = \frac{\sigma^2}{n} \begin{pmatrix} \pi_n^{-1} & 0 \\ 0 & (1-\pi_n)^{-1} \end{pmatrix} = \frac{2\sigma^2}{n} \begin{pmatrix} 1+\frac{D_n}{n} & 0 \\ 0 & 1-\frac{D_n}{n} \end{pmatrix}^{-1},$$

where for a given random vector $\mathbf{u}$ we write $Var[\mathbf{u}] = \mathbf{V}(\mathbf{u})$. If interest is in the joint estimation of (μ_A, μ_B), the D-optimality criterion is usually applied and the goal consists in minimizing

$$\det \mathbf{V}(\hat{\mu}_A, \hat{\mu}_B) = \frac{\sigma^4}{n^2 \pi_n (1-\pi_n)} = \frac{4\sigma^4}{n^2 \left[1 - \left(\frac{D_n}{n}\right)^2\right]}; \tag{2.4}$$

whereas, when the aim is to estimate the difference $\mu_A - \mu_B$, we shall apply the so-called A-optimality and minimize

$$tr\mathbf{V}[\hat{\mu}_A, \hat{\mu}_B] = Var(\hat{\mu}_A - \hat{\mu}_B) = \frac{\sigma^2}{n}\left(\frac{1}{\pi_n} + \frac{1}{1-\pi_n}\right) = \frac{4\sigma^2}{n - \left(\frac{D_n}{\sqrt{n}}\right)^2}. \tag{2.5}$$

A very common problem is testing the hypothesis $H_0 : \mu_A = \mu_B$ versus $H_1 : \mu_A > \mu_B$. Allowing for simplicity $\sigma^2 = 1$ (the case of unknown common variance is analogous (Baldi Antognini, 2008)), the power of the usual z-test of level α is

$$\Phi\left(\frac{\mu_A - \mu_B}{2}\sqrt{n - \left(\frac{D_n}{\sqrt{n}}\right)^2} - z_\alpha\right), \quad \mu_A - \mu_B > 0, \tag{2.6}$$

where $\Phi(z)$ denotes the cumulative distribution function (cdf) of the standard normal and z_α the α-percentile of Φ. Thus, for any sample size n the power is a decreasing function of $|D_n|$ and is maximized when the treatment groups are balanced. The efficiency of a design after n steps with respect to both D-optimality and A-optimality is given by

$$\begin{cases} 1 - \frac{D_n^2}{n^2}, & n \text{ even} \\ \frac{n^2 - D_n^2}{n^2 - 1}, & n \text{ odd} \end{cases} \tag{2.7}$$

and the expected loss of efficiency becomes

$$\begin{cases} E\left[\left(\frac{D_n}{n}\right)^2\right], & n \text{ even} \\ E\left[\frac{D_n^2 - 1}{n^2 - 1}\right], & n \text{ odd.} \end{cases} \tag{2.8}$$

Clearly, the quantities (2.8) are imbalance indicators at step n.

Within the framework of the linear model, and inspired by expressions (2.4) and (2.5), Burman (1996) defines the *loss of precision* induced by lack of balance at step

n as $L_n = n^{-1}D_n^2$, which varies in $[0; n]$. The loss L_n can be interpreted as the equivalent of the number of statistical units on which information is lost due to lack of optimality of the design. Its expectation is

$$\tilde{L}_n = E\left[L_n\right] = E\left[\left(\frac{D_n}{\sqrt{n}}\right)^2\right]. \tag{2.9}$$

The choice of $\tilde{L}_n$ for measuring the lack of balance of randomized rules is a popular one. Atkinson has made intensive simulation studies (see for instance Atkinson (2002)) for comparing several designs in terms of $\tilde{L}_n$. At first sight, (2.9) does not seem a very sensible indicator: the number of lost subjects should be evaluated in relation to n, e.g., by taking into account the expected percentage of lost units

$$E\left[\frac{1}{n}\left(\frac{D_n}{\sqrt{n}}\right)^2\right],$$

but in this case we are driven back to indicator (2.8).

2.3.2 Measures of lack of randomness

There are several ways of measuring allocation randomness or lack thereof. An indicator of lack of randomness measures how far a given allocation rule is from complete randomization, in which at each step the two treatments are allocated with equal probability 1/2, and/or from determinist assignments. A possible measure, originally introduced by Klotz (1978), is the entropy of treatment assignment at step n,

$$-p_n \log_2 p_n - (1 - p_n)\log_2(1 - p_n),$$

where we let $p_n = \Pr\left(\delta_n = 1 \mid \delta^{(n-1)}\right)$ for short. This tends to zero when the allocation is deterministic and is maximized to 1 when $p_n = 0.5$. The probability of deterministic assignments has also been used by some authors (Matts and Lachin, 1988; Berger, 2006).

However, the most popular indicator is a measure of the predictability of the treatment allocations, i.e., the possibility for the experimenter to partially guess the sequence of assignments. Blackwell and Hodges (1957) suggest to measure the degree of predictability of the next step as the probability of a correct guess when the investigator uses an optimal guessing strategy. For designs that assign more probability to the under-represented treatment, this consists of picking the treatment that has been observed fewer times, without preference in case of a tie. The probability of correctly guessing step k conditional on the first $k-1$ steps will be denoted as $\Pr\left(J_k = 1 \mid \delta^{(k-1)}\right)$, where $J_k = 1$ indicates that the k-th assignment is guessed correctly and $J_k = 0$ otherwise. The predictability of the design at step k is measured by

$$\Pr(J_k = 1) = E\left[\Pr\left(J_k = 1 \mid \delta^{(k-1)}\right)\right], \qquad k = 1, \ldots, n.$$

The average predictability after n steps has become known in clinical trials as the *selection bias* SB_n, which is described by the expected percentage of correct guesses up to step n:

$$SB_n = E\left(\frac{1}{n}\sum_{k=1}^{n} J_k\right) = \frac{1}{n}\sum_{k=1}^{n} \Pr(J_k = 1). \tag{2.10}$$

Example 2.3 *For the completely randomized design any strategy is useless, so that at each step* $k \geq 1$ $\Pr(J_k = 1) = 1/2$ *and therefore* $SB_n = 1/2$ *for all* n*, which is the optimal value. Whereas, assuming the Permuted Block Design of size 2*

$$\Pr(J_k = 1) = \begin{cases} 1, & k \text{ even}, \\ \frac{1}{2}, & k \text{ odd}, \end{cases}$$

and thus

$$SB_n = \begin{cases} \frac{3}{4}, & n \text{ even}, \\ \frac{3}{4} - \frac{1}{4n}, & n \text{ odd}. \end{cases}$$

Clearly, if the design is completely deterministic then $\Pr(J_n = 1) = SB_n = 1$ *for every* n*.*

Since for any chosen procedure $1/2 \leq SB_n \leq 1$ for every n, Smith (1984a) has suggested to measure the lack of randomness by the difference between the expected percentage of correct guesses and that of incorrect ones:

$$\tilde{SB}_n = \frac{1}{n}\sum_{k=1}^{n} \Pr(J_k = 1) - \frac{1}{n}\sum_{k=1}^{n} \Pr(J_k = 0) = 2SB_n - 1\,, \tag{2.11}$$

which has the advantage of going from 0 to 1.

2.3.3 Some critical remarks

We end this section making some comments on the proposals we have seen so far.

Remark 2.1 *Both indicators (2.10) and (2.11) have the drawback that at the first stage*

$$\Pr(J_1 = 1) = \frac{1}{2} \quad \Rightarrow \quad SB_1 = \frac{1}{2} \quad \text{and} \quad \tilde{SB}_1 = 0,$$

for any design, since the concept of optimal guessing strategy is useless for the information collected up to step 0, i.e., in absence of information. Furthermore, the probability of correctly guessing the allocation at stage n *depends on the information accrued up to step* $n-1$ *only through the actual imbalance* D_{n-1}*, namely*

$$\Pr(J_n = 1) = E[\Pr(J_n = 1 \mid D_{n-1})],$$

since the optimal strategy consists in picking the under-represented treatment. Thus, in order to avoid i) improper applications of the guessing strategy, and ii) a shifted *time of one step between the evolution of the indicator and that of the design, a suitable correction of the predictability measure at step $k \geq 1$ would be to base it on the probability $Pr(J_{k+1} = 1)$ of guessing correctly the $(k+1)$th allocation, and to define the selection bias indicator as:*

$$SB_n^* = \frac{1}{n} \sum_{k=2}^{n+1} \Pr(J_k = 1). \tag{2.12}$$

Clearly the difference between SB_n and SB_n^* is small for large n, but it does matter in finite sample comparisons.

Remark 2.2 *If the aim is to evaluate the performances of a design over the whole range of sample sizes, indicators like $Var[D_n]$ or $E[|D_n|]$ (up to re-scaling) might be unsuitable, if calculated only for a given sample size n. One should consider the entire sequence $\{E[|D_n|]\}_{n \in \mathbb{N}}$ or $\{Var[D_n]\}_{n \in \mathbb{N}}$. On the other hand, if the design is to be analyzed only for a given n, the measures of average imbalance $n^{-1} \sum_{i=1}^n E[|D_i|]$ or $n^{-1} \sum_{i=1}^n Var[D_i]$ would be preferable. Commonly used indicators of imbalance and randomness like $\tilde{L}_n$ (2.9) and SB_n (2.10) (or, alternatively, (2.11)) are not homogeneous measures. Indeed, $Var[D_n]$ is a local measure of imbalance at step n, while (2.10) is a measure of non-randomness averaged over the first n steps. To evaluate the performance of a design, it is better to match indicators of the same type, e.g.*

$$\tilde{L}_n \quad \textit{and} \quad \Pr(J_{n+1} = 1)$$

or

$$n^{-1} \textstyle\sum_{i=1}^n Var[D_i] \quad \textit{and} \quad SB_n^*.$$

Lastly, it is very hard to derive closed form expressions for measures of imbalance and randomness, due to the generally complex probabilistic structure of the design distribution. An exception is Efron's BCD, for which exact results are available (Markaryan and Rosenberger, 2010). This justifies why in general the behaviour of the above indicators is studied just for large samples, on the basis of asymptotic properties of $\{D_n\}_{n \in \mathbb{N}}$ and $\{|D_n|\}_{n \in \mathbb{N}}$. It is common for authors to evaluate finite sample properties almost exclusively through simulations.

2.4 Classic biased coin designs

After discussing properties of balance and randomness in allocation-adaptive designs from a general point of view, we now proceed to present the designs that have been suggested in the statistical literature, starting from the Biased Coin Design.

2.4.1 The Biased Coin Design

A "biased coin" is a well-known randomization technique that helps neutralize selection bias in sequential experiment for treatment comparison, while keeping the experiment fairly balanced even for all sample sizes. In the original version proposed by Efron (1971), which has already been defined in Chapter 1 and is referred to as the BCD or BCD(p), the allocation of the under-represented treatment is favoured at each step with a prefixed probability $p \in [1/2; 1]$, namely

$$\Pr\left(\delta_{n+1} = 1 \mid \delta^{(n)}\right) = \begin{cases} p & D_n < 0 \\ \frac{1}{2} & D_n = 0\,, \\ 1-p & D_n > 0 \end{cases} \qquad n \geq 1. \tag{2.13}$$

Therefore, at every step the allocation probabilities depend on the sign of the current imbalance, but not on its magnitude. Furthermore, the bias parameter p that controls the degree of randomness is fixed in advance and does not depend on the accrued information, nor on the sample size n. The BCD(p) can be thought to range between CR, the completely randomized design ($p = 1/2$) and PBD_2, the Permuted Block Design ($p = 1$). In order to obtain a valid trade-off between balance and predictability Efron suggests to set $p = 2/3$.

It is easy to show (see Chapter 1) that this is a Markovian design. More precisely, the generating sequence of statistics $\{D_n\}_{n\in\mathbb{N}}$ is an ergodic (i.e. irreducible and positive recurrent) Markov chain. The asymptotic behaviour of the BCD is provided by the steady-state properties of $\{D_n\}_{n\in\mathbb{N}}$, in particular it can be shown that $n^{-1}D_n \to 0$ almost surely as n tends to infinity.

Several extensions of Efron's BCD have been proposed in the literature, all of them fall into two large families: the *Adaptive Biased Coin Designs* (Wei, 1978a) and the *Adjustable Biased Coin Designs* (Baldi Antognini and Giovagnoli, 2004).

2.4.2 The Adjustable Biased Coin Design

Baldi Antognini and Giovagnoli (2004) introduced the Adjustable Biased Coin Design (ABCD), which is an extension of Efron's coin where at each step the probability of selecting the under-represented treatment is a decreasing function of the current difference between the two treatment arms, so that the tendency towards balance is stronger the more we move away from it.

The ABCD is defined by letting

$$\Pr\left(\delta_{n+1} = 1 \mid \delta^{(n)}\right) = F(D_n)\,, \qquad n \geq 1, \tag{2.14}$$

where $F(\cdot) : \mathbb{R} \to [0, 1]$ is a non-increasing function such that

$$F(-x) = 1 - F(x) \qquad \text{for all } x \in \mathbb{R}\,. \tag{2.15}$$

Special cases:

- Efron's BCD(p) is clearly a special case of the ABCD with step function

$$F(x)=\frac{1}{2}+\operatorname{sgn}(x)\left(\frac{1}{2}-p\right); \tag{2.16}$$

- $F(x)=1/2$ for all x gives the CR, while PBD_2 is given by:

$$F(x)=\begin{cases}1 & x\leq -1\\ \frac{1}{2} & x=0\\ 0 & x\geq 1;\end{cases} \tag{2.17}$$

- the BCD With Imbalance Tolerance suggested by Chen (1999)

$$F(x)=\begin{cases}1 & x=-b\\ p & -b+1\leq x\leq -1\\ \frac{1}{2} & x=0\\ 1-p & 1\leq x\leq b-1\\ 0 & x=b\end{cases} \tag{2.18}$$

  where b is a positive integer representing the maximum imbalance tolerated by the investigators;

- the Big Stick Design proposed by Soares and Wu (1983):

$$F(x)=\begin{cases}1 & x=-b\\ \frac{1}{2} & -b+1\leq x\leq b-1\\ 0 & x=b\end{cases} \tag{2.19}$$

  namely a special case of (2.18) with $p=1/2$;

- the Ehrenfest Design (Chen, 2000), that will be further described in Section 2.5:

$$F(x)=\begin{cases}1 & x<-\frac{w}{2}\\ \frac{1}{2}-\frac{x}{w} & -\frac{w}{2}\leq x\leq\frac{w}{2}\,,\\ 0 & x>\frac{w}{2}\end{cases} \tag{2.20}$$

  where w is a positive parameter that plays the same role as b in (2.18) and (2.19).

Rules (2.18), (2.19) and (2.20) are not fully randomized, since the thresholds b and w restrict the support of the process $\{|D_n|\}_{n\in\mathbb{N}}$ by introducing reflecting barriers, which makes some allocations deterministic.

In order to introduce a fully randomized procedure that combines optimal balancing property with a good degree of randomness, Baldi Antognini and Giovagnoli

(2004) have suggested the designs constructed according to the following class of functions, to be denoted by ABCD[$F(a)$]:

$$F_a(x) = \frac{1}{x^a + 1}, \qquad \text{for all } x \geq 1; \tag{2.21}$$

the non-negative parameter a controls the degree of randomness: $a = 0$ gives CR and the design becomes more deterministic as a increases. The rationale behind this choice is to treat the case $|D_n| \leq 1$ as a perfectly balanced design, and to redress the balance only when $|D_n| \geq 2$.

Figure 2.1 shows the allocation probabilities to treatment A for Efron's BCD(2/3) and ABCD[$F(a)$] with $a = 1, 1/2$, $1/4$ and $1/40$ as D_n varies. Due to the symmetric property of these allocation rules the plot deals only with positive values of the imbalance.

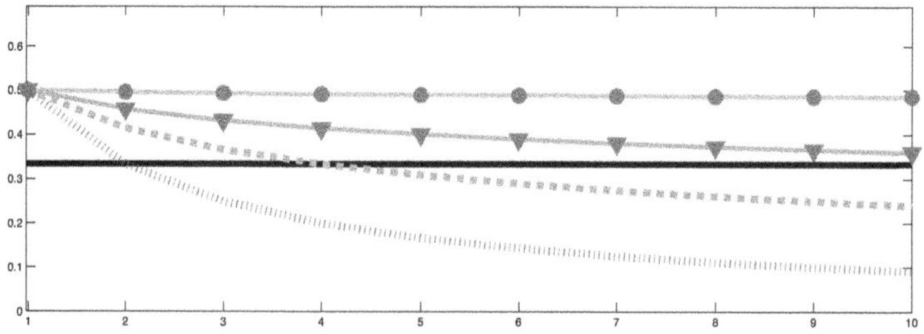

FIGURE 2.1: Allocation probabilities to the under-represented treatment for Efron's BCD(2/3) (solid black) and ABCD[$F(a)$] with $a = 1$ (dotted), 1/2 (dashed), $1/4$ (▼) and $1/40$ (•), as $D_n > 0$ varies.

For instance, if the observed imbalance is $D_n = 4$, ABCD[$F(1)$] assigns the under-represented treatment, i.e., treatment B, to the next subject with probability 0.8, while ABCD[$F(1/2)$] and Efron's coin favour B in the same way, with probability $2/3$; essentially, ABCD[$F(1/40)$] corresponds to CR.

Ergodic random walks are the probabilistic structure underlying the ABCD. Indeed, for any choice of the function $F(\cdot)$, and in particular for Efron's BCD(p), the Markov chain $\{D_n\}_{n \in \mathbb{N}}$ is a time-homogeneous random walk with transition probabilities

$$\Pr(D_{n+1} = j \mid D_n = i) = \begin{cases} F(i) & j = i+1 \\ F(-i) & j = i-1 \end{cases} \quad \text{for all } i \in \mathbb{Z}. \tag{2.22}$$

This chain is irreducible, time-reversible and periodic, with period 2 and, unless $F(\cdot)$ is constant (i.e., the design is CR), the chain is ergodic, so the stationary distribution

$\boldsymbol{\xi}$ exists and is given by the equilibrium equations (Hoel et al., 1972):

$$\begin{aligned} \xi(h) &= \xi(h-1)\lambda_h \qquad \forall h \in \mathbb{Z} \\ \xi(0) &= \left[1+\sum_{s=1}^{\infty}\prod_{h=1}^{s}\lambda_h+\sum_{s=1}^{\infty}\prod_{h=1}^{s}\lambda_{1-h}^{-1}\right]^{-1}, \end{aligned} \tag{2.23}$$

where $\lambda_h = F(h-1)/F(-h)$ for all $h \in \mathbb{Z}$. Unless the design is CR, the sequence $\{\lambda_h\}_{h\in\mathbb{Z}}$ is non-increasing with $\lambda_h = \lambda_{1-h}^{-1}$ for all h, so the stationary distribution $\boldsymbol{\xi}$ in (2.23) is unimodal and symmetric with

$$\xi(h) = \xi(-h), \qquad \text{for all } h \in \mathbb{Z}$$

and 0 represents both the expectation and the mode of $\boldsymbol{\xi}$ with

$$\xi(0) = \left[1+2\sum_{s=1}^{\infty}\prod_{h=1}^{s}\lambda_h\right]^{-1}. \tag{2.24}$$

Clearly, from (2.22) it is easy to show that $\{|D_n|\}_{n\in\mathbb{N}}$ is a homogeneous random walk on the non-negative integers, starting at 0, with

$$\Pr\left(|D_{n+1}| = j \mid |D_n| = i\right) = \begin{cases} F(i) & j = i+1 \\ F(-i) & j = i-1 \end{cases}, \qquad \text{for all } i \geq 1 \tag{2.25}$$

and boundary condition $\Pr\left(|D_{n+1}| = 1 \mid |D_n| = 0\right) = 1$. This chain is periodic and ergodic, with stationary law $\boldsymbol{\xi}^+$ given by

$$\xi^+(0) = \xi(0) \quad \text{and} \quad \xi^+(h) = 2\xi(h) \qquad \forall h \geq 1\,. \tag{2.26}$$

Due to the ergodic property, a direct consequence is that, as n tends to infinity,

$$n^{-\nu}D_n \to 0 \qquad \text{in probability} \quad \text{for all } \nu > 0,$$

and therefore, due to Slutsky's theorem,

$$\lim_{n\to\infty} L_n = \lim_{n\to\infty}\left(\frac{D_n}{\sqrt{n}}\right)^2 = 0 \qquad \text{in probability},$$

so that

$$\lim_{n\to\infty} \tilde{L}_n = \lim_{n\to\infty} E[L_n] = 0.$$

Lastly, we point out that the performance of the ABCD can be assessed for small samples too and not only asymptotically (Baldi Antognini and Giovagnoli, 2004).

2.4.3 Wei's Adaptive Biased Coin Design, Atkinson's D_A-optimum BCD and Smith's Generalized BCD

Since the loss of inferential efficiency induced by a given amount of imbalance decreases as the sample size grows, some authors have introduced extensions of Efron's BCD that take into account the *relative* imbalance, namely $n^{-1}D_n$.

In particular, let $f : [-1, 1] \to [0, 1]$ be a continuous and non-increasing function such that $f(-x) = 1 - f(x)$ for any $x \in [-1; 1]$. Wei (1978a) defines the Adaptive Biased Coin Design by letting:

$$\Pr\left(\delta_{n+1} = 1 \mid \delta^{(n)}\right) = f\left(\frac{D_n}{n}\right), \qquad n \geq 1, \tag{2.27}$$

so that the assignment of the under-represented treatment is favoured increasingly as $n^{-1}|D_n|$ grows.

This is a vast class of procedures based on the probabilistic structure of non-homogeneous Markov chains, whose asymptotic properties have been analyzed in depth. In particular, Wei (1978a) and Smith (1984b) have shown that

$$\lim_{n\to\infty} n^{-1}D_n = 0 \qquad a.s. \tag{2.28}$$

Moreover, due to the continuity of the allocation function $f(\cdot)$, a trivial consequence of (2.28) is that

$$\lim_{n\to\infty} f\left(\frac{D_n}{n}\right) = \frac{1}{2} \qquad a.s.$$

Thus, asymptotically, the Adaptive BCD corresponds to CR and tends to be unpredictable, namely

$$\lim_{n\to\infty} SB_n = \frac{1}{2} \qquad \text{and} \qquad \lim_{n\to\infty} \tilde{SB}_n = 0. \tag{2.29}$$

However, the speed of convergence to balance is very slow and the Markov chain $\{|D_n|\}_{n\in\mathbb{N}}$ diverges as the sample size increases. Indeed, assuming $f(\cdot)$ differentiable at 0, $n^{-1/2}D_n$ is asymptotically normal with

$$n^{-1/2}D_n \to^d N\left(0; \frac{1}{1 - 4f'(0)}\right), \tag{2.30}$$

and therefore:

- the rate of convergence to balance is the same as for the CR, namely of order $n^{-1/2}$;

- since $f(\cdot)$ is non-increasing, then $f'(0) \leq 0$; thus, the asymptotic variance of the Adaptive BCD is lower than that of CR (which is equal to 1).

A trivial consequence of (2.30) is that

$$n^{-1}[1 - 4f'(0)]D_n^2 \to^d \chi_1^2, \tag{2.31}$$

where χ_1^2 is a chi-squared random variable with 1 degree of freedom; thus,

$$L_n \to^d [1-4f'(0)]^{-1}\chi_1^2,$$

and

$$\lim_{n\to\infty} \tilde{L}_n = \frac{1}{1-4f'(0)},$$

since L_n is uniformly integrable; furthermore

$$\lim_{n\to\infty} E[|D_n|] = \infty \qquad \text{and} \qquad \lim_{n\to\infty} Var[D_n] = \infty. \tag{2.32}$$

This is the price that has to be paid in order for the design to become asymptotically as unpredictable as an unbiased coin.

Within this class, a particularly interesting allocation rule is

$$f\left(\frac{D_n}{n}\right) = \frac{\left[1-\left(\frac{D_n}{n}\right)\right]^2}{\left[1-\left(\frac{D_n}{n}\right)\right]^2 + \left[1+\left(\frac{D_n}{n}\right)\right]^2} = \frac{N_{Bn}^2}{N_{An}^2 + N_{Bn}^2}, \tag{2.33}$$

introduced by Atkinson (1982) under the name of D_A-optimum Biased Coin Design. It is inspired by the Wynn–Fedorov sequential construction mentioned in Section 2.1: at step n the allocation probability of treatment $j = A, B$ is proportional to the variance of the predicted difference if we were to allocate that treatment (see Appendix A); Atkinson's design has the advantage of allowing the introduction of covariates (see Chapter 6). Smith (1984a,b) generalized rule (2.33) by letting a non-negative parameter t take the place of the power 2 and obtained the following class of designs:

$$f_t\left(\frac{D_n}{n}\right) = \frac{N_{Bn}^t}{N_{An}^t + N_{Bn}^t}, \tag{2.34}$$

sometimes referred to as the Generalized Biased Coin Design (GBCD). The parameter t controls the degree of randomness: the deterministic component in the design increases as t grows. Special cases are:

- the Completely Randomized design CR ($t = 0$);
- the Generalized Friedman's Urn design (GFU) suggested by Wei (1978b) ($t = 1$), that will be discussed in Section 2.5.1;
- PBD_2 (as $t \to \infty$).

Figure 2.2 illustrates the behaviour of GBCD(t) as t varies.

Remark 2.3 *Under rule (2.34) the second allocation is forced deterministically to balance, i.e., $D_2 = 0$ almost surely, since $f_t(-1) = 1$ and $f_t(1) = 0$; thus, the biased coin mechanism starts only at the third stage and extremely unbalanced allocation sequences, where the same treatment is assigned all the time, are impossible.*

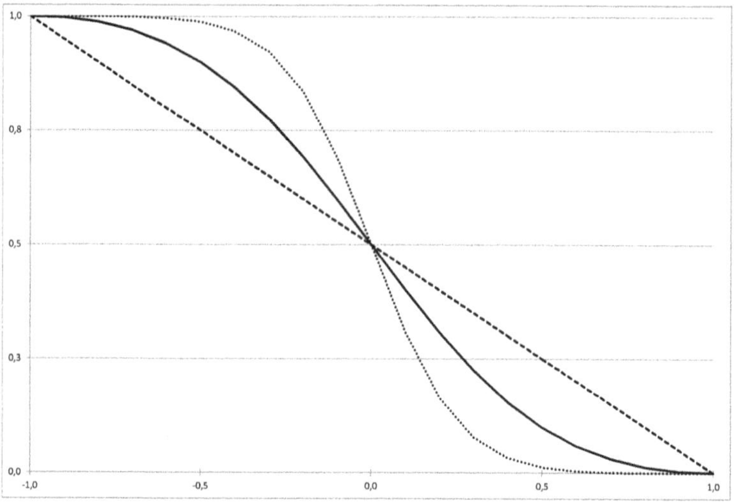

FIGURE 2.2: Allocation probabilities to treatment A for GBCD(t) with $t = 1, 2$ and 3 (dashed, solid and dotted, respectively) as the relative imbalance D_n/n varies.

In order to avoid deterministic assignments, we can modify the GBCD by replacing (2.34) with

$$_pf_t(x) = pf_t(x) + (1-p)f_t(-x)\,, \qquad p \in [1/2; 1] \tag{2.35}$$

which is always randomized; for $p = 1/2$ *the design is completely randomized,* $p = 1$ *corresponds to Smith's GBCD, while for* $t \to \infty$ *rule (2.35) tends to Efron's BCD(p). Figure 2.3 shows the allocation probabilities to treatment A for Atkinson's* D_A*-optimum BCD modified by (2.35) with* $p = 1$ *(i.e., GBCD(*$t = 2$*)), 0.9 and 2/3.*

Remark 2.4 *Since* $f'(0) = -t/2$*, from (2.30) the asymptotic variance of* $n^{-1/2}D_n$ *is inversely proportional to t, with* $\lim_{n\to\infty} Var[n^{-1/2}D_n] = (1+2t)^{-1}$*, and therefore*

$$\lim_{n\to\infty} \tilde{L}_n = \lim_{n\to\infty} \frac{Var[D_n]}{n} = \frac{1}{1+2t}, \tag{2.36}$$

showing the usual inverse relationship between balance and randomness. For instance, assuming Atkinson's D_A*-BCD (namely rule (2.34) with* $t = 2$*) the expected loss converges to* $1/5$.

Parameter $t = -2f_t'(0)$ is an indicator of both balance and predictability.

Finally we stress that, even if the BCD in (2.13) can be regarded as a special case of (2.27) with

$$f\left(\frac{D_n}{n}\right) = \frac{1}{2} + \operatorname{sgn}\left(\frac{D_n}{n}\right)\left(\frac{1}{2} - p\right), \tag{2.37}$$

Efron's procedure does not satisfy the CLT property, since (2.37) is discontinuous at

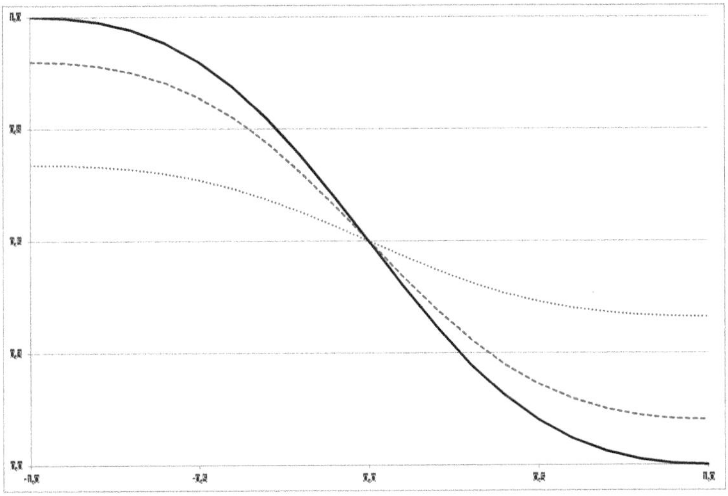

FIGURE 2.3: Allocation probabilities to A for Atkinson's D_A-BCD modified by ${}_pf_2$ in (2.35) with $p = 1, 0.9$ and 2/3 (solid, dashed and dotted lines, respectively) as the relative imbalance D_n/n varies.

0. Indeed, under Efron's coin $n^{-1/2}D_n$ vanishes asymptotically, due to the steady-state property of $\{D_n\}_{n\in\mathbb{N}}$, namely rule (2.13) guarantees a higher order of convergence to balance with respect to Wei's Adaptive BCD. This aspect is crucial in order to understand the different behaviour of these designs.

To explore how these rules work in practice and their drawbacks, consider now three hypothetical trials, illustrated by the scenarios of Table 2.1.

TABLE 2.1: Allocation probabilities to the under-represented treatment for Efron's BCD$(2/3)$ and GBCD(t) with $t = 1$ (GFU), $t = 2$ (Atkinson's D_A-BCD) and $t = 3$, under three different scenarios.

Scenario	n_{An}	n_{Bn}	D_n	BCD$(2/3)$	GFU	D_A-BCD	GBCD(3)
1	3	2	1	0.667	0.6	0.692	0.771
2	51	50	1	0.667	0.505	0.510	0.515
3	60	40	20	0.667	0.6	0.692	0.771

Neither Efron's BCD nor the GBCD distinguish between Scenario #1 (which is balanced since n is odd) and Scenario #3, where treatment A is over-represented with $D_{100} = 20$ (namely the two arms are strongly unbalanced). In the GBCD the tendency towards balance (increasing in t) is stronger for small samples and decreases rapidly as n grows (see Scenarios #1 and #2). On the other hand, since any BCD is insensitive to the magnitude of the imbalance, the allocation will always be driven towards the under-represented treatment with the same probability, so Efron's coin guarantees a higher rate of convergence towards balance.

2.4.4 Comparisons of the Adjustable Biased Coin and Adaptive Biased Coin Designs

The ABCD guarantees a higher rate of convergence to balance with respect to Wei's Adaptive BCD, but the predictability does not vanish asymptotically, since

$$\lim_{n\to\infty} SB_n = 1 + \sum_{s=0}^{\infty}\prod_{x=1}^{s}\frac{F(x-1)}{F(-x)} = \frac{\xi(0)+1}{2},$$

so that

$$\lim_{n\to\infty} \tilde{SB}_n = \xi(0),$$

again stressing the inverse relationship between balance and randomness. For Efron's BCD(p), $\xi(0) = 1 - \{2p\}^{-1}$ and therefore

$$\lim_{n\to\infty} SB_n = 1 - \frac{1}{4p},$$

while for ABCD[$F(a)$] the asymptotic predictability varies between 0 (when $a = 0$, namely under CR) and $1/4$ (as a tends to infinity). Thus, for any choice of a the asymptotic predictability of ABCD[$F(a)$] is no greater than Efron's BCD(2/3), which is equal to $5/8$, and at the same time the loss goes to 0 with the same speed for both rules.

In the ABCD[$F(a)$], the quantity $a/2$ may be regarded as the equivalent of t of Smith's design, since it measures the slope of the function $F_a(x)$ at points $x = 1$ and $x = -1$. So, for a suitable comparison between the ABCD and Smith's design in what follows a will be taken to equal $2t$. In particular for a suitable comparison with Atkinson's D_A-BCD, $a = 1$ has been chosen. Table 2.2 shows the allocation probabilities to the under-represented treatment under ABCD[$F(1)$] and Atkinson's rule as the sample size n and the imbalance D_n vary.

As shown in Table 2.2, for very small samples the tendency towards balance is stronger for Atkinson's D_A-BCD with respect to the ABCD[$F(1)$], while for $n > 10$ the Adjustable BCD allocates the under-represented treatment with higher probabilities. For $n = 100$, the D_A-BCD is close to an unbiased coin, whereas the ABCD forces balance in the same way for any sample size, since it depends only on the observed imbalance. Empty cells in the table mean that the corresponding scenarios are impossible, since $D_n \leq n$ and D_n must have the same parity as n. Also, under Atkinson's rule totally unbalanced allocation sequences are impossible.

Taking now into account a finite sample approach, we compare the performances of Efron's BCD(2/3), Atkinson's D_A-BCD and ABCD[$F(a)$] with $a = 1$ and $1/2$, in terms of imbalance and predictability. The results come from 1000 simulations with $n = 100$.

Starting from balance, Table 2.3 illustrates the same comparison in terms of

TABLE 2.2: Allocation probabilities to the under-represented treatment (B) for ABCD[$F(1)$] and Atkinson's D_A-BCD (within brackets) as n and D_n vary.

	n										
D_n	1	2	3	4	5	6	7	8	9	10	100
1	0.5 (1)		0.5 (0.8)		0.5 (0.69)		0.5 (0.64)		0.5 (0.61)		
2		0.67		0.67 (0.9)		0.67 (0.8)		0.67 (0.74)		0.67 (0.69)	0.67 (0.52)
3			0.75		0.75 (0.94)		0.75 (0.86)		0.75 (0.8)		
4				0.8		0.8 (0.96)		0.8 (0.9)		0.8 (0.85)	0.8 (0.54)
5					0.83		0.83 (0.97)		0.83 (0.93)		
6						0.86		0.86 (0.98)		0.86 (0.94)	0.86 (0.56)
7							0.88		0.88 (0.99)		
8								0.89		0.89 (0.99)	0.89 (0.58)
9									0.9		
10										0.91	0.91 (0.6)

the expected loss $\tilde{L}_n$ in (2.9), while Figure 2.4 shows the performances of the above mentioned procedures by taking into account the average imbalance indicator $n^{-1}\sum_{i=1}^{n} Var[D_i]$.

TABLE 2.3: Expected loss $\tilde{L}_n$ for Atkinson's D_A-BCD, Efron's BCD(2/3) and ABCD[$F(a)$] with $a = 1$ and $1/2$, as n varies.

	n									
	10	20	30	40	50	60	70	80	90	100
D_A-BCD	.214	.201	.196	.212	.218	.206	.210	.220	.208	.203
BCD(2/3)	.315	.202	.142	.098	.088	.063	.056	.050	.047	.045
ABCD[$F(1)$]	.350	.190	.120	.095	.070	.060	.052	.047	.042	.036
ABCD[$F(1/2)$]	.471	.302	.213	.156	.135	.114	.090	.078	.064	.064

As regards the average imbalance, for Atkinson's D_A-BCD the quantity $n^{-1}\sum_{i=1}^{n} Var[D_i]$ tends to diverge as n grows, while the ABCD shows a fast convergence to its asymptotic value. Excluding small sample sizes (we stress that the second assignment of Atkinson's rule is deterministic and this affects the comparisons for starting values of n), the ABCD performs better than Atkinson's rule and this gain increases significantly as n grows. Clearly, as a decreases the imbalance for

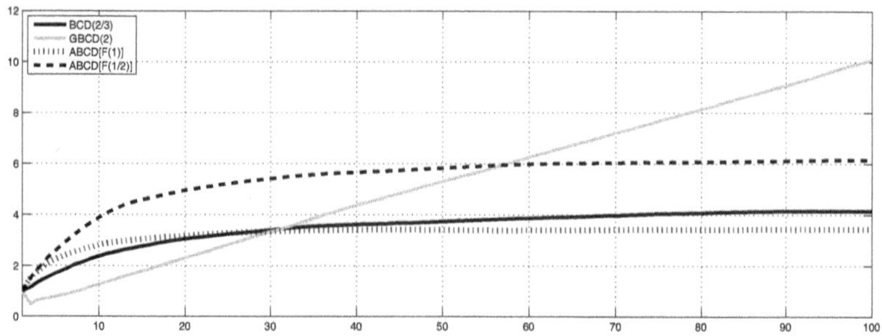

FIGURE 2.4: Average imbalance $n^{-1}\sum_{i=1}^{n} Var[D_i]$ for Atkinson's D_A-BCD (solid grey), Efron's BCD(2/3) (solid black) and ABCD[$F(a)$] with $a = 1$ and $1/2$ (dotted and dashed black lines, respectively) as n varies.

the ABCD[$F(a)$] grows and BCD(2/3) tends to lie between ABCD[$F(1)$] (which seems to be slightly preferable) and ABCD[$F(1/2)$]. The same conclusions can be reached taking into account the expected loss: under D_A-BCD, even from the starting assignments $\tilde{L}_n$ is quite stable around its asymptotic value, i.e., $1/5$, while for the ABCD class of procedures the loss vanishes as n grows, so that for n greater than 30 all the ABCD's perform better than Atkinson's rule.

As regards randomness, Figure 2.5 shows the behaviour of the selection bias SB_n^* in (2.12) for the above mentioned procedures, while Table 2.4 illustrates the same comparison by assuming the probability $Pr(J_{n+1} = 1)$ as a measure of predictability.

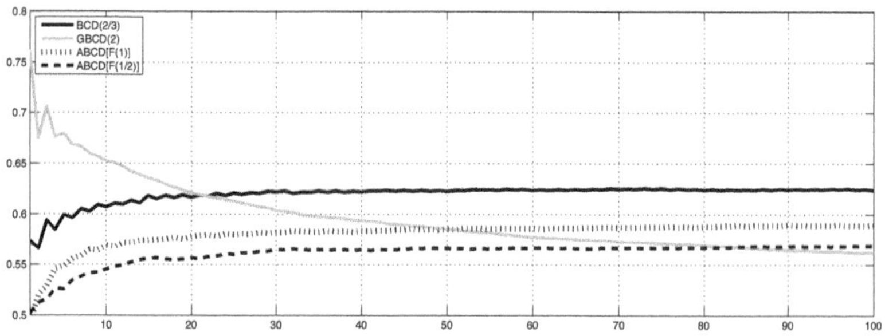

FIGURE 2.5: Selection bias SB_n^* for Atkinson's D_A-BCD (solid grey), Efron's BCD(2/3) (solid black) and ABCD[$F(a)$] with $a = 1$ and $1/2$ (dotted and dashed black lines, respectively) as n varies.

The indicator $\tilde{SB}_n$ is decreasing in n for Atkinson's coin, while it is increasing for the ABCD's. In general, BCD(2/3) is more predictable than all the other procedures, also with respect to ABCD[$F(1)$]. However, as shown in Figure 2.1,

TABLE 2.4: Predictability indicator $Pr(J_{n+1} = 1)$ for Atkinson's D_A-BCD, Efron's BCD(2/3) and ABCD[$F(a)$] with $a = 1$ and $1/2$, as n varies.

	n									
	10	20	30	40	50	60	70	80	90	100
D_A-BCD	.616	.602	.560	.564	.574	.570	.543	.544	.528	.513
BCD(2/3)	.669	.682	.673	.666	.677	.665	.670	.643	.661	.670
ABCD[$F(1)$]	.588	.562	.574	.564	.563	.577	.564	.588	.568	.571
ABCD[$F(1/2)$]	.571	.554	.546	.547	.546	.574	.558	.558	.563	.568

for a given degree of imbalance greater than or equal to 2 the allocation rule of the ABCD[$F(1)$] is always more deterministic than BCD($2/3$), stressing that the behaviour of any procedure is strongly characterized by the definition of the allocation rule when $|D_n| = 1$. If we compare D_A-BCD and ABCD[$F(a)$] on the basis of the sample size, graphical evidence shows that Atkinson's rule performs better than ABCD[$F(a)$] for each choice of a and this gain grows as the sample size increases.

Taking now into account the indicator of predictability $\Pr(J_{n+1} = 1)$, the above conclusions are still valid. The probability of correctly guessing the next allocation is decreasing in n for Atkinson's coin, while under the other procedures it is fairly stable, due to the fast convergence to the stationarity that characterizes the ABCD. Efron's BCD is more predictable than ABCD[$F(a)$] for both choices of a; clearly, the predictability of ABCD[$F(a)$] is decreasing in a. However, as further simulations (omitted here for brevity) have shown, this indicator of predictability is strongly affected by the periodicity of the Markov chain $\{D_n\}_{n\in\mathbb{N}}$, so suitable comparisons between different designs can be usefully performed either for all even (or, alternatively, all odd) sample sizes, but not disregarding the parity of n (as in Figures 2.4 and 2.5).

Remark 2.5 *For all sample sizes, BCD($2/3$) is more predictable than ABCD[$F(1)$] and, at the same time, it is also more unbalanced. Hence, Efron's coin is simultaneously improved upon with respect to both balance and randomness by ABCD[$F(1)$] (see Atkinson (2012)).*

2.5 Urn designs

Urn models were originally introduced and analyzed in the probabilistic literature, see for instance Johnson and Kotz (1977), Gouet (1993), Kotz et al. (2000), Inoue and Aki (2001), Janson (2004), Flajolet et al. (2005), Pouyanne (2005), Flajolet et al. (2006) and Higueras et al. (2006). They are very popular and attractive randomization tools for adaptive designs, due to the simplicity and elegance of their handling, that in some circumstances allows us to derive the asymptotic normality of the allocation proportion of the treatments, as well as the corresponding asymptotic variance. Wei (1977), Wei (1978b, 1979), Schouten (1995), Rosenberger and Lachin (2002), Bai et al. (2002b), Baldi Antognini (2005), Chen (2000, 2006), Muliere et al. (2006a), Zhang et al. (2006), Baldi Antognini and Giannerini (2007) are among the authors who have developed this subject.

In this section we deal with urn models that give rise to allocation-adaptive designs. It is of interest that, for $v = 2$ treatments, most of them are in fact special cases of biased coin designs.

The sequential allocation of two treatments via urn randomization can be intuitively described by the following scheme, usually denoted as the Generalized Pólya Urn (GPU) model. There is an urn containing balls of two different types (colours), one for each treatment. To randomize statistical unit $(n + 1)$, a ball is drawn at random from among all the ones in the urn and if the chosen ball is of type j $(j = A, B)$, then the corresponding treatment will be assigned to the present unit. Let $\mathbf{W}_n = (W_{An}, W_{Bn})$ denote the content vector of the urn, namely W_j represents the number of balls of type j present in the urn after n assignments: the next treatment allocation depends only on the actual urn composition, i.e.,

$$\Pr(\delta_{n+1} = 1 \mid \mathbf{W}_n) = \frac{W_{An}}{W_{An} + W_{Bn}}, \qquad n \geq 1, \tag{2.38}$$

where $W_{An} + W_{Bn}$ is the total number of balls present in the urn at this stage. Then the selected ball of type j is replaced in the urn together with additional $R_n(j, l)$ balls of type l (with $l = A, B$), where negative values are allowed and correspond to removals of balls. Thus, the urn updating process is governed by the *addition* or *replacement* matrix:

$$\mathbf{R}_n = \begin{pmatrix} R_n(A,A) & R_n(A,B) \\ R_n(B,A) & R_n(B,B) \end{pmatrix}, \tag{2.39}$$

which describes the number of balls of type A and B that will be added into the urn, given the current assignment. These operations are repeated at each step and this generates the sequence of allocations. Clearly this scheme can be directly generalized to the case of several treatments (see for instance Bai and Hu (2005)) and can also be described by two different urns, U_A and U_B, standing for the two treatments, each of them containing a given number of balls of just one type: at each step a ball is drawn from either urn at random and if the ball is chosen from U_j, then treatment j is allocated $(j = A, B)$.

Obviously, the evolution of the urn process $\{\mathbf{W}_n\}_{n \in \mathbb{N}}$ - and therefore the behaviour of the associated urn design - is completely specified by the initial urn composition $\mathbf{W}_0$ together with the addition rule $\{\mathbf{R}_n\}_{n \in \mathbb{N}}$. The result below, which is a corollary of Theorem 1.3, highlights the relationship between a sequential urn design and the related urn process and allows us to find urn procedures that converge to any given target proportion of treatment allocations.

Corollary 2.1 *If an urn process $\{\mathbf{W}_n\}_{n\in\mathbb{N}}$ satisfies the following condition*

$$\lim_{n\to\infty}\frac{1}{n}\sum_{i=1}^{n}\frac{W_{Ai}}{W_{Ai}+W_{Bi}}=t \quad a.s. \tag{2.40}$$

then the associated urn design is such that

$$\lim_{n\to\infty}\frac{N_{An}}{n}=t \quad a.s.$$

It goes without saying that, in order to define the allocation probability (2.38), the entries of the initial urn composition vector $\mathbf{W}_0$ and of the addition matrices $\{\mathbf{R}_n\}_{n\in\mathbb{N}}$ do not need to be integers and can be assumed to be real numbers, with suitable constraints on (2.39) to avoid the extinction of balls from the urn. Furthermore, the setting can be extended by letting $\mathbf{W}_0$ and $\{\mathbf{R}_n\}$ be random. In the most general formulation of a GPU model, at each step n each $R_n(j,l)$ $(j,l=A,B)$ may be a function of the accrued information, so that the addition matrix $\mathbf{R}_n$ is random. Several authors refer to this case as the Randomly Reinforced Urn models (see e.g. Muliere et al. (2006a)) or GPU in a random environment (Higueras et al., 2003). For instance, $\mathbf{R}_n$ may depend on the past history by being a function of the sequence of allocations that have been made up to step n. This will lead to a design that is allocation-adaptive. On the other hand, at each step the addition rule may be a function of the observed responses, which leads to a response-adaptive urn design. This latter type will be further studied in Chapter 4.

When the addition matrix is random, the crucial quantity that governs the evolution of the process is the so-called *generating matrix* $\mathbf{H}_n = E\left[\mathbf{R}_n \mid \Im_n\right]$. In particular, if $\mathbf{H}_n=\mathbf{H}$ for all n then the GPU model is said to be *homogeneous* and its asymptotic behaviour (as well as that of the corresponding urn design) depends on the spectral structure of the generating matrix $\mathbf{H}$ (Athreya and Karlin, 1968; Smythe, 1996).

We now proceed to deal with some special urn designs aimed at balancing the allocations of two treatments.

2.5.1 A special class of urn designs

The simplest urn design is when $\mathbf{W}_0=(w/2;w/2)$, with a deterministic and constant adding rule

$$\mathbf{R}_n=\begin{pmatrix} r_{AA} & r_{AB}\\ r_{BA} & r_{BB}\end{pmatrix} \qquad \text{for all } n\geq 1, \tag{2.41}$$

where $w\in\mathbb{R}^+$ and $r_{jl}\in\mathbb{R}$ $(j,l=A,B)$, so that the updating process is the same at every step. Several authors (Wei, 1978b; Chen, 2000, 2006; Baldi Antognini, 2005) have investigated this case in depth. For instance, the case $r_{AA}=r_{BB}=-1$ corresponds to extractions from the urn without replacement. Moreover, special attention has been devoted to the so-called *balanced* urns, namely those such that $r_{AA}+r_{AB}=r_{BA}+r_{BB}=t\geq 0$. At each step t balls are added to the urn and

$$W_{An}+W_{Bn}=w+nt\,, \qquad \text{for all } n\geq 1, \tag{2.42}$$

so that it is sufficient to consider the one-dimensional process $\{W_{An}\}_{n\in\mathbb{N}}$, instead of $\{\mathbf{W}_n\}_{n\in\mathbb{N}}$, where

$$W_{An} = \frac{w + n(r_{AA} - r_{BB} + t) + D_n(r_{AA} + r_{BB} - t)}{2}, \quad \text{for all } n \geq 1. \quad (2.43)$$

The allocation probability (2.38) simply becomes

$$\Pr(\delta_{n+1} = 1 \mid \mathbf{W}_n) = \frac{1}{2} + \frac{n(r_{AA} - r_{BB}) + D_n(r_{AA} + r_{BB} - r)}{2(w + nt)}. \quad (2.44)$$

Clearly, if $t = 0$ the total number of balls is always w at every stage; thus, $\{W_{An}\}_{n\in\mathbb{N}}$ is an irreducible and positive recurrent Markov chain on $\{0, \ldots, w\}$ and (2.44) becomes

$$\Pr(\delta_{n+1} = 1 \mid \mathbf{W}_n) = \frac{1}{2} + \frac{n(r_{AA} - r_{BB}) + D_n(r_{AA} + r_{BB})}{2w}. \quad (2.45)$$

A trivial consequence of Corollary 2.1 for ergodic urn processes is the following:

Corollary 2.2 *Adopting a balanced urn process with* $t = 0$*, the associated urn design is such that*

$$\lim_{n\to\infty} \frac{N_{An}}{n} = \frac{E[W_A]}{w} \quad a.s.$$

where $E[W_A]$ *denotes the ergodic mean of* $\{W_{An}\}_{n\in\mathbb{N}}$.

Thus, in order to obtain an asymptotically balanced urn procedure, the corresponding urn process should be such that $E[W_A] = w/2$.

Special cases:

- *Complete Randomization* corresponds to

$$\mathbf{R}_n = \begin{pmatrix} r & r \\ r & r \end{pmatrix} \quad \text{with } r \geq 0. \quad (2.46)$$

- A very popular urn process is the well-known *Ehrenfest urn* (see Dette (1994), Balaji et al. (2006)), i.e.,

$$\mathbf{R}_n = \begin{pmatrix} -1 & 1 \\ 1 & -1 \end{pmatrix} \quad \text{for all } n \geq 1, \quad (2.47)$$

that has been analyzed in the allocation-adaptive framework by Chen (2000, 2006). At each step one ball is chosen at random without replacement and one ball of the other type is added in the urn. This is a special case of the Adjustable BCD with allocation rule (2.20). By the properties of the stationary distribution of the Ehrenfest process and using an approximation of the k-step transition matrix of $\{W_{An}\}$, Chen has analyzed balance and randomness of the corresponding design, denoted by $EU(w)$, both asymptotically and for small samples.

- *Friedman's urn* (Friedman, 1949) is a special case of the balanced GPU model with deterministic and constant adding matrix. Originally introduced in the context of adaptive designs by Wei (1977), this scheme starts with a even number w of balls equally divided between the two urns, namely $\mathbf{W}_0 = (w/2; w/2)$; at each step one ball is chosen at random and is replaced together with $\beta \geq 0$ additional balls of the other type, i.e.,

$$\mathbf{R}_n = \begin{pmatrix} 0 & \beta \\ \beta & 0 \end{pmatrix}. \tag{2.48}$$

  This scheme was later generalized by Wei (1978b) assuming

$$\mathbf{R}_n = \begin{pmatrix} \alpha & \beta \\ \beta & \alpha \end{pmatrix}, \qquad \alpha, \beta \geq 0, \tag{2.49}$$

  and the associated urn design is usually denoted as $GFU(w; \alpha, \beta)$. From (2.44), there follows

$$\Pr(\delta_{n+1} = 1 \mid \mathbf{W}_n) = \frac{1}{2} - \frac{D_n(\beta - \alpha)}{2[w + n(\alpha + \beta)]}. \tag{2.50}$$

  The parameters α and β represent the weights corresponding to the treatment that has just been assigned and its alternative, respectively. Clearly, for $\beta = \alpha$ we obtain CR, while if $\alpha = w = 0$, starting from an equal allocation probability to either treatment, the design properties do not depend on β. When $\beta > \alpha$, the Generalized Friedman's Urn design $GFU(w; \alpha, \beta)$ is asymptotically equivalent to Wei's Adaptive BCD, due to the fact that the quantity w/n vanishes. In general, $GFU(w; \alpha, \beta)$ is asymptotically balanced, namely

$$\lim_{n \to \infty} \frac{D_n}{n} = 0 \quad a.s.$$

  and furthermore, if $3\beta > \alpha \geq 0$, then as $n \to \infty$

$$\sqrt{n}\left(\frac{N_{An}}{n} - \frac{1}{2}\right) \to^d N\left(0, \frac{\alpha + \beta}{4(3\beta - \alpha)}\right), \tag{2.51}$$

  so the balance is stronger as the value of β/α increases (see also Oden and McIntosh (2006)).

2.5.2 Generalizations of Friedman's urn

A simple extension of Friedman's urn design consists in assuming $\alpha, \beta \in \mathbb{R}$ so that, at each step, we can remove or add a given number of balls from the urn. If $\beta < \alpha$ the treatment which has been assigned in the first allocation will be favoured all the way. Thus, to achieve balance we must consider only the case $\beta \geq \alpha$. In particular, Schouten (1995) has analyzed the special case with $\alpha = -1$ and $\beta \geq 1$

$$\mathbf{R}_n = \begin{pmatrix} -1 & \beta \\ \beta & -1 \end{pmatrix}. \tag{2.52}$$

Another special case is when $\alpha = -\beta \leq 0$, i.e.,

$$\mathbf{R}_n = \begin{pmatrix} -\beta & \beta \\ \beta & -\beta \end{pmatrix}, \tag{2.53}$$

where we assume $\beta \in [0; w/2]$ to avoid the extinction of the balls. Within this extended class, $\beta = 1$ corresponds to the already mentioned Ehrenfest Design. Under (2.53), the process $\{W_{An}\}_{n \in \mathbb{N}}$ is a time-homogeneous and ergodic Markov chain on $\{0, 1, \ldots, w\}$ and the allocation rule (2.50) becomes

$$\Pr(\delta_{n+1} = 1 \mid \mathbf{W}_n) = \frac{1}{2} - \frac{D_n \beta}{w}.$$

Therefore, $\{D_n\}_{n \in \mathbb{N}}$ is a time-homogeneous and ergodic Markov chain on $\{-w/2\beta, \ldots, w/2\beta\}$. This is not surprising, as this procedure is a special case of the Adjustable BCD with a linear allocation function

$$F(x) = \begin{cases} 1 & x < -\frac{w}{2\beta} \\ \frac{1}{2} - \frac{x\beta}{w} & x \in \left[-\frac{w}{2\beta}; \frac{w}{2\beta}\right] \\ 0 & x > \frac{w}{2\beta} \end{cases},$$

and thus is asymptotically balanced (Baldi Antognini, 2005). Further properties of this design can be found in Section 2.4.2.

A further generalization of Friedman's urn has been made by Baldi Antognini and Giannerini (2007) by assuming at every step n a random adding rule of the form:

$$\mathbf{R}_n = \begin{pmatrix} -A_n & A_n \\ B_n & -B_n \end{pmatrix},$$

where A_n and B_n are non-negative random variables with probability distributions depending on the numbers of balls already present in the urn. In particular, the authors provided suitable conditions on the sequences $\{A_n\}_{n \in \mathbb{N}}$ and $\{B_n\}_{n \in \mathbb{N}}$ under which the design is asymptotically normal, namely as $n \to \infty$

$$\sqrt{n}\left(\frac{N_{An}}{n} - \frac{1}{2}\right) \to^d N\left(0; \frac{\sigma^2}{w^2}\right),$$

where σ^2 can be evaluated using a suitable set of orthogonal polynomials (Dette, 1994).

2.6 Some extensions of the biased coin and urn designs of this chapter

In this chapter we have presented classes of adaptive randomized designs that depend on the history of the trial only through the sequence of treatment assignments.

These procedures were originally introduced in the context of comparative clinical trials, where often there are just two treatments and balance is regarded as desirable. However, both the cases of an unbalanced target allocation and of $v > 2$ treatments are also of interest. Several of the designs discussed so far have been generalized in either or both these directions.

Starting from a known target $\pi_A^0 \in (0;1)$ for the allocation proportion of A, the completely randomized design for two treatments can be naturally extended by assigning at each step treatment A with probability π_A^0, namely

$$\Pr\left(\delta_{n+1} = 1 \mid \delta^{(n)}\right) = \pi_A^0 \qquad n \geq 1, \tag{2.54}$$

Efron's coin (2.13) can be generalized by letting

$$\Pr\left(\delta_{n+1} = 1 \mid \delta^{(n)}\right) = \begin{cases} p_2, & \text{if} \quad \pi_n < \pi_A^0 \\ \pi_A^0, & \text{if} \quad \pi_n = \pi_A^0, \\ p_1, & \text{if} \quad \pi_n > \pi_A^0 \end{cases} \qquad n \geq 1, \tag{2.55}$$

with $0 \leq p_1 \leq \pi_A^0 \leq p_2 \leq 1$, where at least one of the inequalities holds strictly. As shown by Baldi Antognini and Zagoraiou (2015), the allocation proportion converges to the chosen target with probability one, i.e.

$$\lim_{n\to\infty} \frac{N_{An}}{n} = \pi_A^0 \qquad a.s.$$

When $p_1 = 1 - p_2$ this corresponds to a special case of the Efficient Randomized Adaptive DEsign (Hu et al., 2009) that will be discussed in Chapter 3. Other authors dealing with this problem are Han et al. (2009) and Kuznetsova and Tymofyeyev (2011, 2012).

Extensions of biased coin designs to the case of $v > 2$ treatments, aimed at achieving a balanced allocation $\pi_j^* = v^{-1}$ for all $j = 1, \ldots, v$ while preserving randomization, are given by Atkinson (1982), Smith (1984a,b) and Wei et al. (1986). For instance, Atkinson (1982) suggests assigning subject $(n+1)$ to treatment j with probability proportional to the generalized variance $d(j,n)$ of the estimated effects j under the linear homoscedastic model

$$\Pr\left(\delta_{j,n+1} = 1 \mid \delta^{(n)}\right) = \frac{d(j,n)}{\sum_{k=1}^{v} d(k,n)}. \tag{2.56}$$

Since $d(j,n) = (n\pi_{jn})^{-1}$ for all $j = 1, \ldots, v$, allocation rule (2.56) becomes

$$\Pr\left(\delta_{j,n+1} = 1 \mid \delta^{(n)}\right) = \frac{\pi_{jn}^{-1}}{\sum_{k=1}^{v} \pi_{kn}^{-1}} = \frac{N_{jn}^{-1}}{\sum_{k=1}^{v} N_{kn}^{-1}}, \tag{2.57}$$

which corresponds to Smith's GBCD($t = 1$) in (2.34) when $v = 2$.

If the interest lies in the estimation of the $v-1$ linear contrasts between the treatment effects, the D_L-optimality criterion is suitable (see Appendix A). Thus, instead of on the quantities $d(j,n)$, the biased coin mechanism can be based on

$$d_L(j,n)=\frac{1}{n}\left(\frac{1}{\pi_{jn}}-1\right), \qquad \forall j=1,\ldots,v$$

and therefore allocation rule (2.56) becomes

$$\Pr\left(\delta_{j,n+1}=1\mid \delta^{(n)}\right)=\frac{d_L(j,n)}{\sum_{k=1}^{v} d_L(k,n)}=\frac{\pi_{jn}^{-1}-1}{\sum_{k=1}^{v}(\pi_{kn}^{-1}-1)}, \tag{2.58}$$

leading to (2.33) in the two-treatment case (i.e., GBCD($t=2$)).

Atkinson's idea was later extended by Ball et al. (1993) in a Bayesian framework, replacing each generalized variance $d(j,n)$ with its monotonic transformation

$$\psi(d(j,n))=\{1+d(j,n)\}^{\frac{1}{\zeta}},$$

where the non-negative parameter ζ controls the degree of randomness. Moreover, Atkinson's rule has been extended to unbalanced target allocations by Wei et al. (1986), Gwise et al. (2008) and Zhao and Weng (2011b), among others.

3

Randomization procedures that depend on the responses

3.1 Introduction

In Chapter 2 we have described adaptive allocation methods based on previous treatment allocations. However, it is intuitively very appealing to choose progressive assignments on the basis of the observed outcomes as well. In some cases, this might prove a necessity, for instance

i) in local optimality problems, when the target allocation is a priori unknown due to its dependence on unknown quantities in the statistical model, such as the parameters, on the functional form of the expected response, etc.;

ii) with ethical concerns about the risks for the subjects involved in the trial, or to economic concern for costs.

Allocations dependent on the accrued data, i.e. "response-adaptive" are possible when the responses are available immediately, but also, with due care, when they are delayed (see Section 1.13). In the present chapter we deal with the response-adaptive designs suggested in the literature for i), while procedures aimed at ii) will be addressed in Chapter 4.

As pointed out in Chapter 1, the experimental information arising from the first n observations is described by the sequence $\Im_n = \{(\delta_1, Y_1), \ldots, (\delta_n, Y_n)\}$, so that a response-adaptive allocation rule will always depend on the past allocations as well, since the accumulated responses refer to specific treatment assignments.

Some examples of response-adaptive rules have been introduced and briefly discussed at the end of Chapter 1. In this chapter we revisit some of the response-adaptive designs of Chapter 1 and introduce new ones. In particular, Sections 3.3-3.5 deal with designs based on sequential estimations, namely the Sequential Maximum Likelihood (SML) design (Melfi and Page, 2000), the Doubly-adaptive Biased Coin Design (D-BCD) (Eisele, 1994; Hu and Zhang, 2004) and the Efficient Randomized Adaptive DEsign (ERADE) (Hu et al., 2009). These are response-adaptive procedures aimed at converging to a given target that depends on the unknown model parameters: starting with n_0 observations on each treatment (usually assigned by restricted randomization), at each step these designs estimate the unknown parameters as well as the target and then modify the next allocation probabilities in order to gradually approach the desired target. In order to describe the properties of these response-adaptive designs, in Section 3.2 we introduce a reparametrization of the exponential family (1.4).

The final section, Section 3.6, deals with Up-and-Down (U&D) procedures. Instead of the comparisons between v qualitative treatments, the underlying framework is a set of ordered treatments, like for example doses of a given drug that might be toxic. The U&Ds are a class of response-adaptive designs aimed at finding which among the treatment levels will produce a desirable pre-specified expected response. Although the U&D algorithm was originally introduced for binary outcomes, we discuss a version that can be applied for any real response variable.

3.2 A more general model for the response

In this section we provide a further asymptotic property of designs converging to a given target allocation. We choose a reparametrization of the exponential family defined in (1.4), that will help in describing the properties of the response-adaptive designs to be considered in Sections 3.3 through 3.5. To avoid cumbersome notation, we restrict ourselves to the case of two treatments A and B. The majority of the asymptotic results hold even in a more general setting and can be easily extended to the case of several treatments (Rosenberger and Lachin, 2002; Hu and Rosenberger, 2006; Hu et al., 2009). We make the usual hypothesis of conditional independence of the outcomes given the treatment assignments and suppose that the responses to either treatment belong to a d-dimensional exponential family, which, conditionally on the treatment, are characterized by the d-dim parameters

$$\gamma_A = E[\boldsymbol{f}(Y) \mid \delta = 1] \quad \text{and} \quad \gamma_B = E[\boldsymbol{f}(Y) \mid \delta = 0] \tag{3.1}$$

where $\boldsymbol{f}$ is a measurable vector function of the responses and we set $\gamma = (\gamma_A^t; \gamma_B^t)^t$.

Usually $\boldsymbol{f}(Y)$ stands for a "natural " sufficient statistic for the chosen model. In the mono-parametric exponential family models, like Bernoulli or or exponential responses, there are no nuisance parameters and $\boldsymbol{f}(Y) = Y$. Otherwise, the presence of several parameters of interest together with nuisance ones can be encompassed by the vector function $\boldsymbol{f}(\cdot)$, in order to express them as functions of the moments of the response distributions. A typical example with $d = 2$ is when the treatment responses are normally distributed with $N(\mu_A; \sigma_A^2)$ and $N(\mu_B; \sigma_B^2)$; in this case if we set $\boldsymbol{f}(Y) = \left(Y; Y^2\right)^t$ then

$$\gamma_A = \left(\mu_A; \mu_A^{(2)}\right)^t \quad \text{and} \quad \gamma_B = \left(\mu_B; \mu_B^{(2)}\right)^t,$$

where $\mu_j^{(2)} = \sigma_j^2 + \mu_j^2$ denotes the second centered moment of the response distribution under treatment j ($j = A, B$). Note that the normal homoscedastic case $\sigma_A^2 = \sigma_B^2$ has the built-in constraint $\mu_A^{(2)} - \mu_A^2 = \mu_B^{(2)} - \mu_B^2$, that must be taken into account in deriving the MLEs.

Under (3.1), at each step n the MLEs of the parameters are

$$\hat{\gamma}_{An} = \frac{\sum_{i=1}^{n} \delta_i \boldsymbol{f}(Y_i)}{\sum_{i=1}^{n} \delta_i} \quad \text{and} \quad \hat{\gamma}_{Bn} = \frac{\sum_{i=1}^{n}(1-\delta_i)\boldsymbol{f}(Y_i)}{\sum_{i=1}^{n}(1-\delta_i)}$$

and the information matrix (conditional on the design) is estimated at step n by

$$\hat{\mathbf{M}}\left(\gamma \mid \pi_n\right) = \mathbf{M}\left(\hat{\gamma}_n \mid \pi_n\right),$$

where $\hat{\gamma}_n = (\hat{\gamma}_{An}^t; \hat{\gamma}_{Bn}^t)^t$. The following result is the analogue of Theorem 1.3 in the present setting.

Theorem 3.1 *Let $\pi^0(\gamma) \in (0;1)$ be a desired target allocation, and assume it to be a continuous function of γ. If the design is such that $\lim_{n\to\infty} \pi_n = \pi^0 = \pi^0(\gamma)$ a.s. then*

- $$\begin{aligned} \lim_{n\to\infty} \mathbf{M}(\hat{\gamma}_n \mid \pi_n) =& \mathbf{M}(\gamma \mid \pi^0(\gamma)) \\ =& diag\left(\pi^0(\gamma)\mathbf{I}_A(\gamma_A), (1-\pi^0(\gamma))\mathbf{I}_B(\gamma_B)\right) \quad a.s. \end{aligned} \tag{3.2}$$

  where $\mathbf{I}_j(\gamma_j)$ is the normalized Fisher information matrix for γ_j associated to a single observation of treatment j (with $j = A, B$), namely

  $$\mathbf{I}_A(\gamma_A) = Var[\boldsymbol{f}(Y_i) \mid \delta_i = 1]^{-1} \quad \textit{and} \quad \mathbf{I}_B(\gamma_B) = Var[\boldsymbol{f}(Y_i) \mid \delta_i = 0]^{-1};$$

- *the ML estimators are strongly consistent*

  $$\lim_{n\to\infty} \hat{\gamma}_n = \gamma \qquad a.s.$$

  and also asymptotically normal with

  $$\sqrt{n}\left(\hat{\gamma}_n - \gamma\right) \to^d N\left(\mathbf{0}; \mathbf{M}^{-1}\left(\gamma \mid \pi^0(\gamma)\right)\right).$$

If $\boldsymbol{f}(\cdot)$ is a vector function, $Var[\boldsymbol{f}(Y_i) \mid \delta_i = 1]$ and $Var[\boldsymbol{f}(Y_i) \mid \delta_i = 0]$ are matrices, and $\mathbf{M}\left(\gamma \mid \pi^0(\gamma)\right)$ in (3.2) is block-diagonal. It is obvious that, when $\boldsymbol{f}(Y_i) = Y_i$, then

$$\begin{aligned} \mathbf{M}\left(\gamma \mid \pi^0(\gamma)\right) =& \text{diag}\left(\frac{\pi^0(\gamma)}{Var[Y_A]}, \frac{1-\pi^0(\gamma)}{Var[Y_B]}\right) \\ =& \text{diag}\left(\pi^0(\gamma) I_A(\gamma_A), (1-\pi^0(\gamma)) I_B(\gamma_B)\right) \end{aligned}$$

is a (2×2)-dim matrix that corresponds to the asymptotic information matrix of the parameters of interest in Theorem 1.3 and $I_j(\gamma_j)$ is the (scalar) normalized information for γ_j associated with a single observation of treatment j ($j = A, B$).

The following definition given in Hu and Rosenberger (2006) applies to adaptive designs for two treatments that converge to a target $(\pi^0(\gamma), 1-\pi^0(\gamma)$.

Definition 3.1 *If the proportion of allocations is asymptotically normal, i.e.,*

$$\sqrt{n}\left(\pi_n - \pi^0(\gamma)\right) \rightarrow^d N(0;\lambda^2), \tag{3.3}$$

the design will be said to be ***asymptotically best*** *for the target $\pi^0(\gamma)$ if the asymptotic variance λ^2 attains its Rao−Cramer lower bound given by* [1]

$$\begin{aligned}\lambda^{2(*)} &= \left(\nabla\pi^0\right)^t \mathbf{M}^{-1}(\gamma \mid \pi^0(\gamma))\left(\nabla\pi^0\right)\\ &= \left(\nabla\pi^0\right)^t diag\left(\frac{\mathbf{I}_A^{-1}(\gamma_A)}{\pi^0(\gamma)};\frac{\mathbf{I}_B^{-1}(\gamma_B)}{1-\pi^0(\gamma)}\right)\left(\nabla\pi^0\right),\end{aligned} \tag{3.4}$$

where $\nabla\pi^0$ denotes the gradient of the function $\pi^0(\gamma)$ with respect to γ.

For any target $\pi^0(\gamma)$, $\lambda^{2(*)}$ in (3.4) is the lowest asymptotic variance of an asymptotically normal treatment allocation proportion converging to that target (it is the same for both treatments). Within the class of such designs, if a response-adaptive procedure attains this lower bound, it cannot be improved in terms of asymptotic variance.

3.3 The Sequential Maximum Likelihood design

There are several circumstances in which the experimenter may wish to choose an experiment that converges to a prescribed target allocation depending on unknown parameters $\boldsymbol{\pi}^0 = \boldsymbol{\pi}^0(\gamma)$. The choice of $\boldsymbol{\pi}^0$ may be motivated by inferential optimality considerations, like the targets of Section 1.7 in Chapter 1, or ethical considerations, like the popular Play-the-Winner target (1.11.2) of Section 1.11.2. In Chapters 4 and 5 several more targets will be introduced, that are motivated by both concerns. The Sequential Maximum Likelihood design (Melfi and Page, 2000) is the simplest adaptively randomized procedure that can be used whenever the desired target depends on some or all the unknown parameters. This design has been hinted at in Section 1.9.1 and here is a full definition.

- We start with a set number n_0 of observations on each treatment in order to provide some initial (non-trivial) estimates of all the parameters involved.
- At each step $n > vn_0$, we estimate the parameters by ML making use of all the data observed up to that step, obtaining $\hat{\gamma}_n^t$, and estimate the target by

$$\hat{\boldsymbol{\pi}}^0 = \boldsymbol{\pi}^0(\hat{\gamma}_n).$$

[1] In the first edition of Hu and Rosenberger (2006), the calculation of $\lambda^{2(*)}$ in some instances is incorrect.

- Then we assign the next treatment with probabilities given by the current estimate of the target, namely

$$\Pr\left(\delta_{n+1,j} = 1 \mid \delta^{(n)}, Y^{(n)}\right) = \pi_j^0(\hat{\gamma}_n), \quad \text{for all } j = 1, \ldots, v;\ n > vn_0. \tag{3.5}$$

3.3.1 Asymptotic properties and drawbacks of the SML design

We show that

Theorem 3.2 *If $\pi^0(\gamma) \in (0;1)$ and is continuous in γ, then the SML design converges almost surely to the target, namely*

$$\lim_{n\to\infty} \boldsymbol{\pi}_n = \boldsymbol{\pi}^0(\gamma) \quad a.s. \tag{3.6}$$

Proof *First of all we point out that the assumption of Lemma 1.1 is satisfied by the allocation rule (3.5), so that $\lim_{n\to\infty} N_{jn} = \infty$ $a.s.$ for $j = 1, \ldots, v$. Hence the strong consistency of the ML estimators in the present setting (see Section 1.8.2), so that by continuity*

$$\lim_{n\to\infty} \boldsymbol{\pi}^0(\hat{\gamma}_n) \to \boldsymbol{\pi}^0(\gamma) \quad a.s.$$

The rest of the proof follows directly from Theorem 1.1.

For two treatments A and B from Theorem 3.1 there follows that

$$\begin{aligned} \lim_{n\to\infty} \mathbf{M}(\hat{\gamma}_n \mid \pi_n) &= \mathbf{M}(\gamma \mid \pi^0(\gamma)) \\ &= \text{diag}\left(\pi^0(\gamma)\mathbf{I}_A(\gamma_A), (1-\pi^0(\gamma))\mathbf{I}_B(\gamma_B)\right) \quad a.s. \end{aligned} \tag{3.7}$$

and, as well as consistency, we get the asymptotic normality of the ML estimators

$$\sqrt{n}\left(\hat{\gamma}_n - \gamma\right) \to^d N\left(\mathbf{0}; \mathbf{M}^{-1}\left(\gamma \mid \pi^0(\gamma)\right)\right).$$

Moreover, Eisele (1994),Eisele and Woodroofe (1995) and Hu and Zhang (2004) have proved the following version of the Central Limit Theorem for the allocation proportions of the SML design:

$$\sqrt{n}\left(\pi_n - \pi^0(\gamma)\right) \to^d N(0; \lambda^2_{SML}), \tag{3.8}$$

with

$$\lambda^2_{SML} = \pi^0(\gamma)\left(1-\pi^0(\gamma)\right) + 2\left(\nabla\pi^0\right)^t \mathbf{M}^{-1}\left(\gamma \mid \pi^0(\gamma)\right)\left(\nabla\pi^0\right). \tag{3.9}$$

The SML design is a natural extension of CR, and also of procedure (2.54), to the case of target allocations depending on model parameters. Since the target is unknown and is estimated step by step using the available information, there is a further variability in the asymptotic variance of the allocation proportions given by the quadratic form $\left(\nabla\pi^0\right)^t \mathbf{M}^{-1}\left(\gamma \mid \pi^0(\gamma)\right)\left(\nabla\pi^0\right)$ in (3.9). In the special case when the target π^0 is known, i.e., it does not depend on the model parameters, $\nabla\pi^0 = \mathbf{0}$. No recurrent estimation of the target is needed: the SML design trivially becomes randomization rule (2.54), namely at each step the allocation of treatment A is a Bernoulli random variable $Be\left(\pi^0\right)$; the asymptotic variance of the allocation proportion is simply $\pi^0\left(1-\pi^0\right)$.

To summarize:

- when adopting the SML design, the allocation probabilities depend only on the current estimate of the target and are not affected by the actual allocation proportions; the SML forces the assignments of each treatment in the same way, independently of whether its current allocation proportion is close to (or far from) the target;
- asymptotically, the SML randomizes the treatments according to the corresponding target allocations;
- from the asymptotic normality (3.8), the convergence of the allocation proportion to the chosen target is slow, also due to the high asymptotic variance in (3.9), so that for small samples the SML design may generate large departures from the target.

3.3.2 An example

Assume that the responses of the two treatments have exponential distributions $Exp\left(\theta_A\right)$ and $Exp\left(\theta_B\right)$, so that $\boldsymbol{\gamma}^t = (\theta_A, \theta_B)$. The optimal target allocation to A when the criterion is A-optimality is

$$\pi^*(\theta_A;\theta_B) = \frac{\theta_A}{\theta_A+\theta_B}$$

(see Table 1.1). The associated SML design is

$$\Pr\left(\delta_{n+1}=1|\boldsymbol{\delta}^{(n)},\mathbf{Y}^{(n)}\right) = \frac{\hat{\theta}_{An}}{\hat{\theta}_{An}+\hat{\theta}_{Bn}}, \qquad \forall n \geq 2n_0$$

which, by Theorem 1.3, turns out to be asymptotically A-optimal for unconditional inference. Applying Theorem 3.2,

$$\lim_{n\to\infty} \pi_n = \frac{\theta_A}{\theta_A+\theta_B} \qquad a.s.$$

and the MLEs $\hat{\theta}_{An}$ and $\hat{\theta}_{Bn}$ are strongly consistent and asymptotically normal, with asymptotic variance-covariance matrix

$$\mathbf{M}^{-1}\left(\boldsymbol{\gamma} \mid \pi^*(\boldsymbol{\gamma})\right) = \text{diag}\left(\theta_A(\theta_A+\theta_B);\theta_B(\theta_A+\theta_B)\right),$$

since $I_j(\gamma_j) = \theta_j^{-2}$ for $j = A, B$. Thus, the allocation proportion to treatment A is asymptotically normal with

$$\sqrt{n}\left(\pi_n - \frac{\theta_A}{\theta_A+\theta_B}\right) \to^d N\left(0;\frac{3\theta_A\theta_B}{(\theta_A+\theta_B)^2}\right),$$

since

$$\pi^*(\theta_A;\theta_B)\,(1-\pi^*(\theta_A;\theta_B)) = \frac{\theta_A\theta_B}{(\theta_A+\theta_B)^2}$$

and

$$\nabla\pi^* = \left(\frac{\theta_B}{(\theta_A+\theta_B)^2}; \frac{-\theta_A}{(\theta_A+\theta_B)^2}\right)^t.$$

3.4 The Doubly-adaptive Biased Coin Design

Doubly-adaptive biased coin designs (D-BCDs) are an important family of response-adaptive randomization procedures: they consist of a modification of SML designs, aimed at driving the assignments towards the given target faster than the SML. They make use of some measure of "dissimilarity" between the actual treatment allocation proportions and the current estimate of the target. The rationale consists in favouring at every step the allocation of the treatment whose current allocation proportion is smaller than the current estimate of its target in such a way that the smaller the allocation proportion is, the greater is the probability of assigning the treatment.

The idea goes back to Eisele (1994) who introduced it in the case of two treatments under the regular exponential family model, but was later generalized by Hu and Zhang (2004) to several treatments and more complex response models. The following is a slight modification of Eisele's original definition of the Doubly-adaptive Biased Coin Design.

Consider a function $g : [0,1]^2 \to [0,1]$ such that

C1) $g(x;y)$ is continuous on $(0;1)^2$;

C2) $g(x;x) = x$;

C3) $g(x;y)$ is decreasing in x and increasing in y on $(0;1)^2$.

The function $g(x;y)$ stands for the assignment probability, x stands for the current allocation proportion and y for the current estimated target. After a pilot stage with n_0 observations on each treatment for initial estimation, the D-BCD is defined by

$$\Pr\left(\delta_{n+1} = 1 \mid \delta^{(n)}, Y^{(n)}\right) = g\left(\pi_n; \pi^0(\hat{\gamma}_n)\right), \quad \text{for all } n > 2n_0. \tag{3.10}$$

The D-BCD will drive the allocation proportion towards the target, since from conditions C2) and C3), when $x > y$ then $g(x;y) \geq y$ so if the current allocation proportion of treatment A is greater than the estimated target, the probability of assigning this treatment is lower than the estimated target and vice versa. Clearly, we get the SML design by letting $g(x;y) = y$ for any $x \in [0;1]$.

Although not necessary for the convergence properties of the design, the following further condition

C0) $g(x;y) = 1 - g(1-x; 1-y)$ for all $x, y \in (0;1)^2$

guarantees that A and B are treated symmetrically.

The above definition of the D-BCD includes several well-known adaptive designs, but not all of them. For instance:

- when the target does not depend on the unknown parameters, e.g., when $\pi^0 = 1/2$, then $g(x;y)$ is constant in y and the design is allocation-adaptive. The CR design, Wei's Adaptive BCD and rule (2.54) can be regarded as special cases of the D-BCD, by taking $g(x;y) = 1/2$, $g(x;y) = f(x)$ and $g(x;y) = \pi_A^0$ respectively. However, Efron's BCD is excluded since the allocation function is discontinuous, thus contradicting Condition C1).
- the ABCD is also excluded, since it corresponds to a sequence of allocation rules $\{g_n(x;y)\}_{n\geq 1}$, with $g_n(x;y) = F(n(2x-1))$, instead of a fixed $g(\cdot\,;1/2)$.

The convergence of the Doubly-adaptive Biased Coin Designs is ensured under some conditions on the target:

Proposition 3.1 *If $\pi^0(\gamma) \in (0;1)$ and is continuous in γ, then the D-BCD converges to the target, namely*

$$\lim_{n\to\infty} \pi_n = \pi^0(\gamma) \quad a.s.$$

The result is a consequence of Theorem 1.2 by letting $t(\boldsymbol{y}) = \pi(\gamma)$. The almost sure convergence to the target of the ABCD too can be proved by means of Theorem 1.2, that does not require the continuity of the allocation rule g and also allows for a sequence of different allocation rules.

Under further conditions on the randomization function g and the target allocation $\pi^0(\gamma)$, the asymptotic normality of the D-BCD design can be proved.

Theorem 3.3 *(Eisele, 1994) Assuming C1) through C3), the hypothesis of Proposition 3.1 and the following further regularity conditions:*

C4) $g(x;y)$ is differentiable[2] *in both arguments, with bounded partial derivatives, and such that*

$$\frac{\partial g(x;y)}{\partial x}\Big|_{x=y=\pi^0(\gamma)} \neq 0, \tag{3.11}$$

C5) $\pi^0(\gamma)$ is a twice continuously differentiable function,

then

$$\sqrt{n}\left(\pi_n - \pi^0(\gamma)\right) \to^d N\left(0;\lambda^2\right), \tag{3.12}$$

where

$$\lambda^2 = \frac{\pi^0(\gamma)\left(1-\pi^0(\gamma)\right)}{1-2d_x} + \frac{2d_y^2(\nabla\pi^0)^t \mathbf{M}^{-1}\left(\gamma \mid \pi^0(\gamma)\right)(\nabla\pi^0)}{(1-d_x)(1-2d_x)}, \tag{3.13}$$

[2]This differentiability condition is very restrictive (Melfi et al., 2001), so that Hu and Zhang (2004) introduced an alternative condition that requires bounded partial derivatives only around the target and avoids (3.11).

and

$$d_x = \frac{\partial g(x;y)}{\partial x} \mid_{x=y=\pi^0(\gamma)} \quad \text{and} \quad d_y = \frac{\partial g(x;y)}{\partial y} \mid_{x=y=\pi^0(\gamma)} .$$

Recalling that the allocation function g must be decreasing in x and increasing in y, then $d_x \leq 0$ and $d_y \geq 0$, so the asymptotic variance of the design decreases when the allocation function $g(x;y)$ tends to be strongly decreasing in x and quite flat in y locally around the target.

Within the D-BCD class, Hu and Zhang (2004) suggest the following family of allocation functions

$$g_\alpha(x;y) = \frac{y(y/x)^\alpha}{y(y/x)^\alpha + (1-y)[(1-y)/(1-x)]^\alpha}, \tag{3.14}$$

with

$$g_\alpha(0;y) = 1 \quad \text{and} \quad g_\alpha(1;y) = 0, \tag{3.15}$$

where the non-negative parameter α controls the degree of randomness of each allocation: if α is near zero, the dependence of the randomization function on the current allocation proportion is very weak and the design will tend to resemble the SML design; whereas as α grows, the allocation tends to be forced deterministically to the estimated target and for $a \to \infty$ rule (3.14) corresponds to the design considered by Robbins et al. (1967). Note however that, for the limit cases $\alpha = 0$ and $\alpha \to \infty$, conditions (3.15) do not hold.

The D-BCD (3.14) guarantees in general a smaller asymptotic variance of the allocation proportions, although the rate of convergence to the target is the same as for the SML design, namely of order $\sqrt{n}$. To see this, it is easy to check that

$$d_x = -\alpha < 0 \quad \text{and} \quad d_y = 1 + \alpha > 1, \tag{3.16}$$

so that for any chosen target allocation the asymptotic variance in (3.13) is always smaller than that of the SML design in (3.9), as shown in the following example.

Example 3.1 *In the setting of the example of Section 3.3.2, i.e., responses with exponential distributions and A-optimal target, we now look at the D-BCD with allocation function g_α in (3.14). The asymptotic variance of the allocation proportion is*

$$\frac{\theta_A\theta_B}{(\theta_A+\theta_B)^2}\left(\frac{3+2\alpha}{1+2\alpha}\right),$$

which is always less than (or equal to) $3\theta_A\theta_B(\theta_A+\theta_B)^{-2}$, since $\alpha \geq 0$. In particular, if we set $\alpha = 1$ the asymptotic variance of the D-BCD is around 55% of that of the SML design.

Example 3.2 *When the target is a priori known, the Doubly-adaptive Biased Coin Design becomes allocation-adaptive and if $\pi^0 = 1/2$ the D-BCD corresponds to Wei's Adaptive BCD defined in (1.17) with $g(x;1/2) = f(2x-1)$ (provided condition C0) holds true). Clearly $\nabla\pi^0 = \mathbf{0}$ and thus the asymptotic variance of $\sqrt{n}\pi_n$*

is $\{4(1-2d_x)\}^{-1}$, *which corresponds to (1.30) by recalling that* $D_n/n = 2\pi_n - 1$ *and*

$$\frac{\partial g(x;1/2)}{\partial x}\mid_{x=1/2} = 2f'(0).$$

For the D-BCD with allocation function g_α as in (3.14), it is evident because of (3.16) that the randomization parameter α controls the behaviour of the allocation function around the target. The asymptotic variance (3.13) of the allocation proportion

$$\frac{\pi^0(\gamma)\left(1-\pi^0(\gamma)\right)}{1+2\alpha} + (\nabla\pi^0)^t\mathbf{M}^{-1}\left(\gamma \mid \pi^0(\gamma)\right)(\nabla\pi^0)\left(\frac{2(1+\alpha)}{1+2\alpha}\right) \quad (3.17)$$

is strictly decreasing in α and, as $\alpha \to \infty$, attains the Rao–Cramer lower bound $\lambda^{2(*)}$ in (3.4).

Example 3.3 *When the responses to treatment* j *follow a normal distribution* $N(\mu_j;\sigma_j^2)$ *with* $j = A, B$, *the A-optimal target is Neyman's allocation:*

$$\pi^*(\gamma_A;\gamma_B) = \frac{\sigma_A}{\sigma_A+\sigma_B}.$$

As shown in Section 3.2, in order to express the target as a function of the first two centered moments of the normal distribution we let $\boldsymbol{f}(Y) = \left(Y;Y^2\right)^t$, *so that*

$$\pi^*(\gamma_A;\gamma_B) = \frac{\sqrt{\mu_A^{(2)}-\mu_A^2}}{\sqrt{\mu_A^{(2)}-\mu_A^2}+\sqrt{\mu_B^{(2)}-\mu_B^2}}.$$

The asymptotic variance in (3.13) of the D-BCD becomes (see Hu and Zhang (2004) for details)

$$\lambda^2 = \frac{\sigma_A\sigma_B}{(\sigma_A+\sigma_B)^2}\left[\frac{1}{1-2d_x}\left(1+\frac{d_y^2}{1-d_x}\right)\right]. \quad (3.18)$$

If we use the allocation function g_α *in (3.14),*

$$\lambda^2 = \frac{\sigma_A\sigma_B}{(\sigma_A+\sigma_B)^2}\frac{2+\alpha}{1+2\alpha}, \quad (3.19)$$

which is always smaller than the asymptotic variance of the SML design:

$$\frac{2\sigma_A\sigma_B}{(\sigma_A+\sigma_B)^2}.$$

Furthermore, as $\alpha \to \infty$, *the asymptotic variance of* g_α *in (3.19) attains its Rao–Cramer lower bound*

$$\lambda^{2(*)} = \frac{\sigma_A\sigma_B}{2(\sigma_A+\sigma_B)^2}.$$

Another proposal for the allocation function of the D-BCD is (Baldi Antognini and Zagoraiou, 2012; Baldi Antognini et al., 2012):

$$g(x;y) = \frac{G\left[D(x;y)G^{-1}(y)\right]}{G\left[D(x;y)G^{-1}(y)\right] + G\left[D(1-x;1-y)G^{-1}(1-y)\right]}, \tag{3.20}$$

where $G : \mathbb{R}^+ \to \mathbb{R}^+$ is a continuous and strictly increasing function, while $D(x;y) : (0;1)^2 \to \mathbb{R}^+$ stands for a measure of dissimilarity between the actual allocation proportion x and the current estimate of the optimal target y; D is assumed to be a continuous function, decreasing in x and increasing in y, with $D(x;x) = 1$. For example, if $D(x;y) = 1$ for all $(x,y) \in (0,1)^2$, then (3.20) corresponds to the SML design, while if we let $G(t) = t$ and $D(x;y) = (y/x)^\alpha$, one obtains $g_\alpha(x;y)$ in (3.14). If we set $D(x;y) = y/x$ and

$$G(z) = \frac{2}{\sqrt{\pi}} \int_0^z e^{-t^2} dt \qquad \text{(i.e. the so-called } \textit{error function} \text{ Erf}(z));$$

this leads to

$$\tilde{g}(x;y) = \frac{G\left[\frac{y}{x}G^{-1}(y)\right]}{G\left[\frac{y}{x}G^{-1}(y)\right] + G\left[\frac{1-y}{1-x}G^{-1}(1-y)\right]}. \tag{3.21}$$

Otherwise, letting $G(t) = t$ and $D(x;y) = 1-(x-y)$, rule (3.20) becomes

$$\dot{g}(x;y) = \frac{y[1-(x-y)]}{y[1-(x-y)] + (1-y)[1-(y-x)]}. \tag{3.22}$$

In order to compare the properties of the allocation functions g_α in (3.14), $\tilde{g}$ in (3.21) and $\dot{g}$ in (3.22), Table 3.1 shows the probabilities of assigning treatment A when both the target estimate and the allocation proportion vary.

In general, the allocation rule g_α is strongly affected by the value of x, i.e., by the current allocation proportion: if one treatment has almost never been assigned then g_α allocates it in a deterministic way, independently of the value of the corresponding target allocation y. Furthermore, g_2 tends to be highly deterministic, while $\tilde{g}$ and $\dot{g}$ force the allocations towards the target only when needed, guaranteeing at the same time a greater degree of randomness than g_α. To summarize, the allocation rule g_α is characterized by a strong deterministic component in the assignments, which has a clear impact in terms of asymptotic variance, as the following example shows.

Example 3.4 *In the same setting as Example 3.3, if we adopt the randomization function $\dot{g}$ in (3.22), then*

$$d_x = \frac{-2\sigma_A\sigma_B}{(\sigma_A+\sigma_B)^2} \qquad \textit{and} \qquad d_y = 1 + \frac{2\sigma_A\sigma_B}{(\sigma_A+\sigma_B)^2}$$

and, by (3.18), the asymptotic variance of the allocation proportion is

$$\lambda^2 = \frac{2\sigma_A\sigma_B}{(\sigma_A+\sigma_B)^2}\left[\frac{1+\frac{\sigma_A\sigma_B}{(\sigma_A+\sigma_B)^2}}{1+4\frac{\sigma_A\sigma_B}{(\sigma_A+\sigma_B)^2}}\right].$$

TABLE 3.1: Probabilities of allocating treatment A for the D-BCD with allocation functions $\tilde{g}$ in (3.21), $\dot{g}$ in (3.22) and g_α in (3.14) with $\alpha = 1$ and 2.

x	y	g_1	g_2	$\tilde{g}$	$\dot{g}$
$\to 0$	0.1	1.000	1.000	0.537	0.120
$\to 0$	0.3	1.000	1.000	0.653	0.443
$\to 0$	0.5	1.000	1.000	0.792	0.750
$\to 0$	0.7	1.000	1.000	0.916	0.930
$\to 0$	0.9	1.000	1.000	0.990	0.994
0.2	0.1	0.047	0.022	0.051	0.083
0.2	0.3	0.424	0.557	0.407	0.344
0.2	0.5	0.800	0.941	0.735	0.650
0.2	0.7	0.956	0.995	0.897	0.875
0.2	0.9	0.997	0.999	0.988	0.981
0.4	0.1	0.018	0.003	0.025	0.056
0.4	0.3	0.216	0.151	0.227	0.260
0.4	0.5	0.600	0.692	0.585	0.550
0.4	0.7	0.891	0.966	0.859	0.813
0.4	0.9	0.992	0.999	0.984	0.964
0.6	0.1	0.008	0.001	0.016	0.036
0.6	0.3	0.109	0.034	0.141	0.188
0.6	0.5	0.400	0.308	0.415	0.450
0.6	0.7	0.784	0.850	0.773	0.740
0.6	0.9	0.982	0.997	0.975	0.944
0.8	0.1	0.003	$\simeq 0$	0.012	0.019
0.8	0.3	0.044	0.005	0.103	0.125
0.8	0.5	0.200	0.059	0.265	0.350
0.8	0.7	0.577	0.443	0.593	0.656
0.8	0.9	0.953	0.979	0.949	0.917

Thus, for any choice of $\alpha > 1/2$ the D-BCD with allocation rule g_α guarantees a smaller asymptotic variance than that of $\dot{g}$, due to the fact that

$$2\left[\frac{\sigma_A\sigma_B}{(\sigma_A+\sigma_B)^2}\right] \leq 2\left(\frac{1}{4}\right) \leq \frac{1}{2}.$$

As shown by Baldi Antognini and Zagoraiou (2012), the dissimilarity measure $D(x;y)$ can be discontinuous, so that the allocation rule (3.20) becomes discontinuous too. In this case the asymptotic properties of the D-BCD cannot be applied; however, procedure (3.20) corresponds to a special case of the Reinforced Doubly-adaptive Biased Coin Design (to be discussed in Chapter 6 for the case of covariates), another design converging almost surely to any desired target allocation.

Example 3.5 *Set $G(t) = t$ and*

$$D(x;y) = \begin{cases} 1+\rho, & x<y \\ 1, & x=y, \\ 1-\rho, & x>y \end{cases} \qquad \textit{with } \rho \in [0,1),$$

then the allocation function (3.20) becomes

$$\ddot{g}(x;y)=\begin{cases}\frac{y(1+\rho)}{y(1+\rho)+(1-y)(1-\rho)}, & x<y\\ y, & x=y.\\ \frac{y(1-\rho)}{y(1-\rho)+(1-y)(1+\rho)}, & x>y\end{cases} \tag{3.23}$$

As a consequence of Theorem 1.2 we can prove the convergence of this design to any chosen target, namely

Proposition 3.2 *If $\pi^0(\gamma)\in(0;1)$ is continuous in γ, then adopting the allocation rule (3.23)*

$$\lim_{n\to\infty}\pi_n=\pi^0(\gamma)\quad a.s.$$

3.5 The Efficient Randomized Adaptive Design

As shown previously, in the response adaptive setup the D-BCD plays the same role with respect to the SML design as Wei's Adaptive BCD with respect to CR in the allocation-adaptive framework. In fact, D-BCD and SML designs are both asymptotically normal, but the tendency of the D-BCD to force the allocations on the basis of the proportion of treatment assignments already observed induces a reduction of the asymptotic variance of the design. As is well known, asymptotic normality determines slow convergence (the rate is $\sqrt{n}$). This is related to the continuity of the allocation function around the target; it is due to the fact that, asymptotically, the estimated target $\hat{\pi}_n^0$ converges almost surely to the chosen one π^0 and since $g(x;y)$ is jointly continuous with $g(x;x)=x$, the D-BCD tends to assign treatment A with probability $\simeq\pi^0$ infinitely often. This is the exactly the same behaviour as Wei's Adaptive BCD when the chosen target is the balanced one.

In the same spirit as Efron's BCD, Hu et al. (2009) introduced the Efficient Randomized Adaptive DEsigns (ERADE) in order to improve the convergence to the chosen target. This too is a class of response-adaptive procedure aimed at converging to any desired target $\pi^0(\gamma)$, that is a continuous function of the unknown model parameters. In particular, the ERADE assigns treatment A to the $(n+1)$th patient with probability

$$\Pr\left(\delta_{n+1}=1\mid\delta^{(n)},Y^{(n)}\right)=\begin{cases}\rho\pi^0(\widehat{\gamma}_n), & \pi_n>\pi^0(\widehat{\gamma}_n)\\ \pi^0(\widehat{\gamma}_n), & \pi_n=\pi^0(\widehat{\gamma}_n),\\ 1-\rho\left[1-\pi^0(\widehat{\gamma}_n)\right], & \pi_n<\pi^0(\widehat{\gamma}_n)\end{cases} \tag{3.24}$$

where $\rho\in[0;1)$ is a randomization parameter;. When $\rho=0$ the design becomes the deterministic one suggested by Robbins et al. (1967), while as ρ grows the allocations are more randomized and for $\rho\to1$ the ERADE tends to the SML design. When the desired target is the balanced one, i.e., $\pi^0(\gamma)=1/2$, the choice $\rho=2(1-p)$

corresponds to Efron's BCD(p) (e.g., ERADE with $\rho = 2/3$ reduces to Efron's BCD(2/3)).

The convergence of the ERADE is ensured by the following corollary of Theorem 1.2.

Proposition 3.3 *If $\pi^0(\gamma) \in (0;1)$ is continuous in γ, the ERADE converges almost surely to the target, namely*

$$\lim_{n\to\infty} \pi_n = \pi^0(\gamma) \quad a.s.$$

Proof *As a function of $x = \pi_n$ and $y = \pi^0(\widehat{\gamma}_n)$ the allocation rule of the ERADE can be rewritten as follows*

$$\varphi^{ERADE}(x;y) = \begin{cases} \rho y, & \text{if } x > y, \\ y, & \text{if } x = y, \\ 1-\rho(1-y), & \text{if } x < y, \end{cases}$$

which has a single generalized downcrossing $t(y) = y$. Therefore the almost sure convergence follows immediately from the continuity of the target.

Assuming that $\pi^0(\gamma)$ is a twice continuously differentiable function of γ, Hu et al. (2009) show that

$$\sqrt{n}\left(\hat{\gamma}_n - \gamma\right) \to^d N\left(\mathbf{0}; \mathbf{M}^{-1}\left(\gamma \mid \pi^0(\gamma)\right)\right)$$

and

$$\sqrt{n}\left(\pi_n - \pi^0(\gamma)\right) \to^d N\left(0; \lambda^{2(*)}\right), \tag{3.25}$$

where $\lambda^{2(*)}$ is the Rao–Cramer lower bound for the asymptotic variance of a design targeting $\pi^0(\gamma)$. This establishes the asymptotic efficiency of the ERADE for any choice of the randomization parameter $\rho \in [0;1)$. After some simulation studies, the authors recommend to choose $\rho \in (0.4; 0.7)$ in order to obtain a valid trade-off between randomization and efficiency.

3.6 The Up-and-Down design

Up-and-Down is the name of a type of adaptive designs used in dose-response studies, e.g., in toxicology and pharmacology, and in industrial applications. The aim is to investigate the effect on a response variable Y of a stimulus, for instance the dosage of a drug: given the level $x \in \mathbb{R}$, the expected value $E[Y \mid x]$ is assumed to be a strictly increasing function $Q(x)$ of the stimulus and we are interested in finding which value of the input $x_{(\Gamma)}$ will produce a prescribed mean response Γ. In toxicology, for instance, the responses are binary and the probability of positive response (toxicity) is assumed to be an increasing function of the given dose level; the aim is estimating the dose associated to a pre-specified probability of positive response. Classical examples are the median $LD(50)$, i.e., the dose that is lethal for 50% of the population under trial, or the maximum tolerated dose (MTD) of Phase I clinical trials. As a rule, the response curve $Q(x)$ is unknown and the problem is the search for the unknown target level $x_{(\Gamma)}$.

In the experimental setting, there are a finite number of pre-specified values of x that can be tried (the treatments) so in this case the treatments are ordered. The set of available treatment levels, in increasing order, can be denoted by $\mathcal{D} = \{d_0, \ldots, d_M\}$ (not necessarily equally spaced). We write $Q(d_j) = Q_j$ ($j = 0, 1, \ldots, M$) for short. In the Up-and-Down (U&D) method, at each step one or more observations are taken using a given treatment level and according to the response, at the next step the treatment is either a) increased by one level, or b) decreased by one level, or c) maintained at the same level.

The very first version of the U&D algorithm for binary responses, proposed by von Bekesy (1947) and Dixon and Mood (1948) in order to target $LD(50)$, was deterministic: the experiment simply consisted in observing one unit at a time and decreasing the treatment level if the response was positive, increasing it if negative. Later, a randomization mechanism of the biased coin type was introduced by Derman (1957) and Durham and Flournoy (1994) to cope with the search for a quantile of Q, i.e., $x_{(\Gamma)} = Q^{-1}(\Gamma)$ corresponding to a value of Γ $(0 < \Gamma < 1)$ different from 0.5, where $Q^{-1}(p) = \inf\{x : Q(x) \geq p\}$. Since then, U&D has been the object of a large amount of investigation by various authors (Durham et al., 1997; Giovagnoli and Pintacuda, 1998; Ivanova et al., 2003; Ivanova and Flournoy, 2006; Bortot and Giovagnoli, 2005; Gezmu and Flournoy, 2006; Baldi Antognini et al., 2008; Baldi Antognini and Crimaldi, 2006). We are going to define a U&D design for general outcomes and a given target, which clusters the treatment allocations around the target level. Methods of inference for U&D designs will also be discussed.

3.6.1 Definition and properties of U&D designs

We shall assume the expected response $Q(x)$ to be known when x is a minimum $(x = d_0)$ or a maximum $(x = d_M)$, so that these values are of no interest for our experiment. We can either observe just one unit at each step or more than one, but we assume that the response Y is a scalar, e.g., the sum or the mean of the observations from the group of units. We denote by $\mathcal{Y}$ the range of Y and put $\inf \mathcal{Y} = a$ and $\sup \mathcal{Y} = b$. Set also $\mathcal{I} = [a; b]$. We assume that $Q(\cdot)$ is strictly increasing.

Let X_n denote the treatment level applied at step n and let Y_n be the corresponding outcome. To randomize the design, at each step we define the probabilities of increasing or decreasing the treatment by one level in terms of the outcomes. More precisely, we choose two functions from $\mathcal{Y}$ into $[0, 1]$ – the *generating functions* $\alpha(\cdot)$ and $\beta(\cdot)$ of the design – such that:

- $\alpha(y) + \beta(y) \leq 1$ for all $y \in \mathcal{Y}$;
- $\alpha(\cdot)$ is decreasing and $\beta(\cdot)$ is increasing (not necessarily strictly);

- $\lim_{y\to a}\alpha(y) \geq \lim_{y\to a}\beta(y)$ and $\lim_{y\to b}\alpha(y) \leq \lim_{y\to b}\beta(y)$.

U&D Rule

Choose a starting point $x_1 \in \mathcal{D}$. At each step $n \geq 1$, given the treatment $X_n = d_j$ ($j = 0, 1, \ldots, M-1$) the next level will be chosen as follows

$$\begin{aligned} X_{n+1} &= d_{j+1} \text{ with probability } \alpha(Y_n), \\ X_{n+1} &= d_{j-1} \text{ with probability } \beta(Y_n), \\ X_{n+1} &= d_j \quad \text{with probability } 1-\alpha(Y_n)-\beta(Y_n), \end{aligned} \tag{3.26}$$

and at the extremes d_0 and d_M,

$$\begin{aligned} \Pr\left(X_{n+1} = d_1 \mid X_n = d_0\right) &= 1, \\ \Pr\left(X_{n+1} = d_{M-1} \mid X_n = d_M\right) &= 1. \end{aligned} \tag{3.27}$$

This design is response-adaptive and Markovian and it is easy to show that the sequence $\{X_n\}_{n\geq 1}$ of the design points is a random walk on the state space $\mathcal{D}$, with transition probabilities

$$\begin{aligned} p_j &= \Pr(X_{n+1} = d_{j+1} \mid X_n = d_j) = E[\alpha(Y_n) \mid X_n = d_j] \\ q_j &= \Pr(X_{n+1} = d_{j-1} \mid X_n = d_j) = E[\beta(Y_n) \mid X_n = d_j] \\ r_j &= \Pr(X_{n+1} = d_j \mid X_n = d_j) = 1 - p_j - q_j, \end{aligned}$$

for $j = 1, \ldots M-1$, and reflecting barriers $p_0 = q_M = 1$.

Hence the Markov chain $\{X_n\}_{n\geq 1}$ is irreducible and positive recurrent. If $r_j > 0$, it is aperiodic with a unique stationary distribution $\boldsymbol{\xi}^t = (\xi(d_1), \ldots, \xi(d_M))$ given by the equilibrium equations

$$\begin{aligned} \xi(d_j) &= \xi(d_{j-1})\frac{p_{j-1}}{q_j} = \xi(d_{j-1})\frac{E[\alpha(Y) \mid d_{j-1}]}{E[\beta(Y) \mid d_j]}, \quad j = 1, \ldots, M \quad (3.28) \\ \xi(d_0) &= \left[1 + \sum_{j=1}^{M}\prod_{i=1}^{j}\frac{p_{i-1}}{q_i}\right]^{-1}. \end{aligned}$$

Lemma 3.1 *When the following condition is satisfied,*

U) the sequence $\{p_j\}$ is decreasing and the sequence $\{q_j\}$ is increasing,

the stationary distribution $\boldsymbol{\xi}$ is unimodal with mode d_K, where

$$K = \max\{j \in \{2, \ldots, M-1\} \textit{ such that } p_{j-1} > q_j\}.$$

The proof of this lemma can be found in Durham and Flournoy (1994) and Giovagnoli and Pintacuda (1998).

What assumptions ensure that condition U) of Lemma 3.1 holds true?

Lemma 3.2 *A sufficient condition on the statistical model to ensure U) is that Y be stochastically increasing with respect to its expectation $E[Y \mid \cdot]$.*

Proof *In this case* $E[Y \mid x] = Q(x)$ *is a strictly increasing function of* x*, so* Y *is stochastically increasing in* x*. Then* $\alpha(\cdot)$ *decreasing and* $\beta(\cdot)$ *increasing imply that* $E[\alpha(Y) \mid x]$ *is a decreasing function of* x *and* $E[\beta(Y) \mid x]$ *is increasing in* x *(see Ross (1996)).*

The requirement of Lemma 3.2 is very strong, however it is satisfied by common distributions, like the binary, binomial, Poisson, exponential and homoscedastic normal cases.

Under condition U), for any pre-specified Γ, the design can be made to target the unknown $x_{(\Gamma)}$ such that $Q(x_{(\Gamma)}) = \Gamma$, as follows.

Proposition 3.4 *For any given* $\Gamma \in \mathcal{I}$*, let the generating functions* $\alpha(\cdot)$ *and* $\beta(\cdot)$ *be chosen so that*

$$E[\alpha(Y) \mid Q(x) = \Gamma] = E[\beta(Y) \mid Q(x) = \Gamma] \qquad (\text{"targeting condition"}) \quad (3.29)$$

then

$$d_{K-1} < x_{(\Gamma)} \leq d_{K+1}, \qquad (3.30)$$

where $x_{(\Gamma)}$ *is the target. This means that mode* d_K *of the stationary distribution is within one level from the target.*

We now turn the attention to the asymptotic behaviour of the design. Let $\pi_{jn} = N_{jn}/n$ be the proportion of allocations to d_j after n steps; from the Strong Law of Large Numbers for Markov chains we have

$$\lim_{n \to \infty} \pi_{jn} = \xi(d_j) \qquad a.s. \qquad \forall\, j = 0, 1, \ldots, M. \qquad (3.31)$$

Thus, for n sufficiently large the mode of the empirical distribution $\boldsymbol{\pi}_n = (\pi_{0n}, \pi_{1n}, \ldots, \pi_{Mn})$ is a valid candidate as an estimator of $x_{(\Gamma)}$. Some of its properties are discussed in Giovagnoli and Pintacuda (1998).

3.6.2 A special case: Binary responses

The U&D was first introduced in the case when the responses are binary and at each stage only one unit is observed, so that $\mathcal{Y} = \{0, 1\}$ and $\mathcal{I} = [0; 1]$. The Bernoulli distribution $Be(Q(x))$ satisfies condition U). Without loss of generality put $Q(d_0) = 0$ and $Q(d_M) = 1$, since other cases can be reduced to this setup by applying a straightforward linear transformation of $Q(\cdot)$. The transition probabilities are

$$\begin{aligned} p_j &= \alpha(0)(1 - Q_j) + \alpha(1)Q_j, \\ q_j &= \beta(0)(1 - Q_j) + \beta(1)Q_j, \\ r_j &= 1 - p_j - q_j. \end{aligned}$$

The U&D rule (3.26) is the one proposed in Giovagnoli and Pintacuda (1998) if we set

$$\begin{aligned} \alpha(0) &= \alpha > \alpha(1) = \alpha', \\ \beta(0) &= \gamma' < \beta(1) = \gamma, \end{aligned} \qquad (3.32)$$

with $\max\{\alpha+\gamma', \alpha'+\gamma\} \leq 1$ and $\max\{\alpha', \gamma'\} \leq \min\{\alpha, \gamma\}$.

Condition (3.29) becomes

$$\frac{\alpha(0)-\alpha(1)}{\alpha(0)-\alpha(1)+\beta(1)-\beta(0)} = \Gamma.$$

Among the special cases is the DF rule introduced in Chapter 1

$$\begin{aligned} \alpha(0) &= \min\left(\frac{\Gamma}{1-\Gamma}, 1\right), \quad \alpha(1) = 0 \\ \beta(0) &= 0, \quad \beta(1) = \min\left(\frac{1-\Gamma}{\Gamma}, 1\right) \end{aligned} \tag{3.33}$$

which satisfies condition (3.29).

Example 3.6 *Consider the function $Q(x) = x^2$ in $[0,1]$ to be the probability of positive response. Let the set $\mathcal{D}$ of available treatment levels be the sequence of values $0, 0.1, 0.2, \ldots$ up to 1. We seek the quantile that corresponds to probability $\Gamma = 0.2$ of positive response, which means $x_{(0.2)} = 0.45$. With the DF rule the transition probabilities p, q, r and the stationary distribution are given in Table 3.2.*

TABLE 3.2: Transition probabilities p, q, r and stationary distribution of the DF rule.

Treatment level	$Q(x)$	p	q	r	ξ
0.0	0.00	0.25	0.00	0.75	0.000
0.1	0.01	0.25	0.01	0.74	0.012
0.2	0.04	0.24	0.04	0.72	0.076
0.3	0.09	0.23	0.09	0.68	0.203
0.4	0.16	0.21	0.16	0.63	0.289
0.5	0.25	0.19	0.25	0.56	0.243
0.6	0.36	0.16	0.36	0.48	0.126
0.7	0.49	0.13	0.49	0.38	0.041
0.8	0.64	0.09	0.64	0.27	0.008
0.9	0.81	0.05	0.81	0.14	0.001
1.0	1.00	0.00	1.00	0.00	0.000

The stationary distribution has a peak at $x = 0.4$, which is a good approximation of the quantile of interest.

3.6.3 A special case: Binomial responses

Essentially, this is the Randomized Group U&D introduced in Baldi Antognini et al. (2008): at each step n we observe binary responses from m units and the probabilities of increasing or decreasing the treatment level are functions of the number Y_n of observed successes. The binomial distribution $Bin(m, Q(x))$ satisfies U). The properties of the algorithm depend on the choice of the generating functions $\alpha(\cdot)$ and $\beta(\cdot)$, and several possible choices are discussed in Baldi Antognini et al. (2008). For instance with the following stepwise functions

$$\alpha(y) = \begin{cases} \alpha, & y \leq s \\ 0, & \text{otherwise} \end{cases} \quad \text{and} \quad \beta(y) = \begin{cases} \beta, & y \geq t \\ 0, & \text{otherwise} \end{cases} \quad y \in [0, m],$$

where s and t are integers $0 \leq s < t \leq m$, we obtain a randomized version of the Group U&D by Gezmu and Flournoy (2006), namely at each step the level is increased with probability $\alpha > 0$ if the number of positive responses is $\leq s$, whereas it is decreased with probability $\beta > 0$ if the number of positive responses is $\geq t$; s and t must satisfy the targeting condition

$$\alpha \sum_{k=0}^{s} \binom{m}{k} \Gamma^k (1-\Gamma)^{m-k} = \beta \sum_{k=t}^{m} \binom{m}{k} \Gamma^k (1-\Gamma)^{m-k}. \tag{3.34}$$

Gezmu and Flournoy (2006)'s Group U&D experiments are obtained when $\alpha = \beta = 1$, and therefore are deterministic. One drawback is that, for a given target probability Γ, there might not exist integers m, s and t such that condition (3.34) is satisfied. Randomizing the experiment with α and β overcomes this difficulty.

Example 3.7 *One example of Group U&D design is the experiment with $m = 3$, $s = 0$ and $t = 2$ suggested by Storer (2005), similar to the so-called standard method adopted in Phase I clinical trials (Korn et al., 1994). By substituting these values in (3.34) and solving with respect to Γ we get $\Gamma = 0.347$, thus Storer's experiment is targeted approximately on $\Gamma = 34\%$.*

Example 3.8 *The so-called geometric U&D or "k-in-a-row"(KR), introduced by Wetherill et al. (1966) and revisited by Oron and Hoff (2009), also falls within this type of experiment. Assuming binary responses, a KR experiment starts at an arbitrary level, and then moves one level down following each positive response, or one level up when observing k consecutive negative responses, all at the same level. We can think of it as a Group U&D with $m \geq k$ units in each group and $s = 0$, $t = 1$, except that when a decision about increasing or decreasing the level has already been reached the remaining units in the group are not observed, with obvious advantages. It is easy to see from (3.34) that the KR design is associated to probability $\Gamma = 1 - 2^{-1/k}$. For $k = 2, 3$ and 4, the target quantiles are approximately $x_{(0.293)}$, $x_{(0.206)}$ and $x_{(0.159)}$, respectively.*

3.6.4 A special case: Normal responses

Assume that for each unit the distribution of the response Y given x is normal with constant variance $N(Q(x), \sigma^2)$. This model satisfies condition U). If at each step we observe m units, Y can be replaced by the sample mean, with distribution

$N(Q(x), \sigma^2/m)$. For a given $\epsilon > 0$, set

$$\alpha(y) = \alpha I_{(-\infty, \Gamma-\epsilon]}(y),$$
$$\beta(y) = \alpha I_{[\Gamma+\epsilon, +\infty)}(y) .$$

In other words, we increase the level with probability α when we observe a value $\leq \Gamma - \epsilon$ and decrease it with the same probability if we observe $y \geq \Gamma + \epsilon$. The targeting condition (3.29) becomes

$$\Phi\left(\frac{-\epsilon}{\sigma}\right) = 1 - \Phi\left(\frac{\epsilon}{\sigma}\right),$$

which is always satisfied $\forall \alpha \in (0; 1]$. The transition probabilities are

$$\begin{aligned} p_j &= E[\alpha(Y_n) \,|\, X_n = d_j] = \alpha\Phi\left(\frac{\Gamma - \epsilon - Q_j}{\sigma}\right), \\ q_j &= \Pr(X_{n+1} = d_{j-1} \,|\, X_n = d_j) = \alpha\left[1 - \Phi\left(\frac{\Gamma + \epsilon - Q_j}{\sigma}\right)\right], \\ r_j &= \Pr(X_{n+1} = d_j \,|\, X_n = d_j) = 1 - p_j - q_j. \end{aligned} \tag{3.35}$$

Example 3.9 *Let* $x \in [0; 1]$ *and*

$$Y|x \sim N\left(1 + \log\frac{x}{1-x}; 0.09\right).$$

Let the set $\mathcal{D}$ *of available treatment levels be* $0.1, 0.2, 0.3, \ldots$ *up to* 0.9*, giving vales of the response function ranging roughly between* 0 *and* 2*. Let the level of interest correspond to an expectation* $\Gamma = 1.3$*, which implies* $x_{(1.3)} = 0.67$*, and choose* $\epsilon = 0.1$*. The algorithm moves away from the very low levels with probability practically equal to 1. The transition probabilities p and q and the stationary distribution are given in Table 3.3. The peak of the stationary distribution is between* 0.6 *and* 0.7*.*

3.6.5 Asymptotic inference for Up-and-Down experiments

Several estimators of the target have been considered for U&D experiments. A non-parametric one is the mode of the empirical distribution, as seen before. On the other hand, it is also common to assume a parametric model for the function $Q(\cdot)$, and consider estimating the unknown target by maximum likelihood. For example Durham et al. (1997) assumed the two-parameter logistic model or a location-scale model for the binary response curve and analyzed the maximum likelihood estimators under the DF design (Durham and Flournoy, 1994), showing that the MLEs retain the asymptotic normality property. For any given Γ, if the generating functions $\alpha(\cdot)$ and $\beta(\cdot)$ satisfy the assumption of Proposition 3.4, by (3.30) the target $x_{(\Gamma)}$ lies in a neighborhood of the mode d_K of the stationary distribution $\boldsymbol{\xi}$ so the asymptotic precision of the MLEs at the target is highest. Furthermore, the precision increases as the peakedness of the stationary distribution rises (see also (3.37 below). Thus, for n

TABLE 3.3: Transition probabilities and stationary distribution of U&D with normal responses.

Treatment levels	$Q(x)$	p	q	ξ
0.1	0.05	0.9999	0.0000	0.0000
0.2	0.40	0.9962	0.0004	0.0000
0.3	0.63	0.9708	0.0052	0.0003
0.4	0.82	0.8950	0.0274	0.0104
0.5	1.00	0.7475	0.0912	0.1020
0.6	1.18	0.5318	0.2277	0.3348
0.7	1.37	0.2878	0.4575	0.3891
0.8	1.60	0.0901	0.7497	0.1494
0.9	1.95	0.0060	0.9677	0.0139

sufficiently large the maximum likelihood method provides a valid estimation procedure. Stylianou and Flournoy (2002) have proposed an estimate of the target based on a linearly interpolated isotonic regression; adopting the DF, they illustrate the performance of the proposed estimator by simulations.

Some authors prefer to estimate the whole curve $Q(\cdot)$ in a non-parametric way, and thus obtain an estimate of the target. Supposing that the response Y at a given treatment level $X = x$ has distribution belonging to the exponential family (1.4) with $\theta_x = E[Y \mid X = x] = Q(x)$, at each step n, the current MLE $\hat{Q}_{jn}$ of Q_j is the sample mean

$$\hat{Q}_{jn} = \frac{S_{jn}}{N_{jn}}, \qquad \text{for } j = 0, \ldots, M, \tag{3.36}$$

where S_{jn} denotes the sum of the observation that are allocated to d_j up to n. From Theorem 1.3 the following asymptotic results are easily established.

Proposition 3.5 *Let* $\hat{\boldsymbol{Q}}_n = \left(\hat{Q}_{0n}, \ldots, \hat{Q}_{Mn}\right)$ *be the MLEs of* $\boldsymbol{Q} = (Q_0, \ldots, Q_M)$ *under a U&D experiment. Then as* $n \to \infty$

- $\hat{\boldsymbol{Q}}_n \to \boldsymbol{Q} \qquad a.s.$
- $\sqrt{n}\left(\hat{\boldsymbol{Q}}_n - \boldsymbol{Q}\right) \to^d N(0; \boldsymbol{\Sigma})$,

where

$$\boldsymbol{\Sigma} = diag\left(\frac{Var[Y|X = d_j]}{\xi(d_j)}\right)_{j=0,\ldots,M}. \tag{3.37}$$

It must be pointed out that this is not an efficient approach. Unless n is very large, in a U&D experiment some of the treatment levels will not be observed at all, and some others will be observed a very limited number of times, thus making the estimation of the whole curve $Q(x)$ impossible or very approximate.

3.6.6 On the asymptotic optimality of U&D experiments

A fully satisfactory criterion for comparing U&D experiments is at present still to be found. Ideally, we would like to place a very large fraction of the available observations around the unknown target; for U&D designs with the same target $x_{(\Gamma)}$, an asymptotic criterion has been suggested which compares the *peakedness* around $x_{(\Gamma)}$ of the corresponding stationary distributions.

Definition 3.2 *(Giovagnoli and Pintacuda, 1998) Given two U&D experiments* $U\&D^{(1)}$ *and* $U\&D^{(2)}$*, both targeted on the same* $x_{(\Gamma)}$*, the stationary distribution* $\boldsymbol{\xi}^{(1)}$ *of* $U\&D^{(1)}$ *is said to be more peaked around* $x_{(\Gamma)}$ *than the stationary distribution* $\boldsymbol{\xi}^{(2)}$ *of* $U\&D^{(2)}$ *if, for all* $j = 1, \ldots, M-1$,

$$\begin{aligned} Q_j < \Gamma \ \textit{implies} \ \frac{\xi^{(1)}(d_j)}{\xi^{(1)}(d_{j-1})} &\geq \frac{\xi^{(2)}(d_j)}{\xi^{(2)}(d_{j-1})} \quad \textit{and} \\ Q_j \geq \Gamma \ \textit{implies} \ \frac{\xi^{(1)}(d_{j+1})}{\xi^{(1)}(d_j)} &\leq \frac{\xi^{(2)}(d_{j+1})}{\xi^{(2)}(d_j)}. \end{aligned} \tag{3.38}$$

Given the asymptotic normality of the design, another criterion of interest is its asymptotic variance, which affects the speed of convergence to stationarity.

Example 3.10 *For binary responses and the U&D rule defined by Giovagnoli and Pintacuda (1998) show that, all else being the same, the choice* $\alpha(1) = \beta(0) = 0$ *improves the peakedness of the algorithm around the target. With this choice, writing* $\alpha(0) = \alpha$ *and* $\beta(1) = \beta$ *for short, the targeting condition becomes*

$$\frac{\alpha}{\alpha+\beta} = \Gamma,$$

so that

$$\beta = \left(\frac{1-\Gamma}{\Gamma}\right)\alpha.$$

As to the best choice of α *according to condition (3.38), it can be shown to be*

$$\alpha = \min\left(\frac{\Gamma}{1-\Gamma}, 1\right),$$

i.e., the DF rule. Furthermore, Bortot and Giovagnoli (2005) have shown that the algorithm DF can in most cases be regarded as optimal among all U&D rules for binary responses with respect to the asymptotic variance of the treatment level frequencies and to the speed of convergence to stationarity. A simulation study has confirmed the optimality of the DF rule, which however converges very slowly, but has also highlighted the dependence of the precision of the estimates of $x_{(\Gamma)}$ *on the starting value of the algorithm.*

3.6.7 Extensions of U&Ds

Attempts have been made to extend the U&D method in several ways.

U&D algorithms are very myopic rules insofar as the decision on the next level is made to depend only on the most recent outcome. An alternative idea is a second-order Markovian experiment which in theory allows greater flexibility. Second-order U&D designs were defined by Bortot and Giovagnoli (2005) in the case of binary responses: the next step of the algorithm is based on the outcome of the last two observations, instead of making use of just the most recent value. More in detail: assume $0 < \Gamma < 0.5$. With the DF rule, when a negative response is observed the treatment level is increased with probability α. A natural extension is to increase the level with probability α_0 if the previous observation is also negative and probability α_1 if it is positive. The level is always decreased when a positive response is observed, as in the DF design. Second-order U&Ds share some desirable properties with the first-order ones, in particular the convergence of the empirical frequencies to a stationary distribution with mode around the quantile of interest. Comparison of some second-order U&D's with the optimal first-order ones, both as regards the stationary distribution from a theoretical viewpoint, and the precision of quantile estimates via simulation, have shown that higher order experiments can, with a suitable choice of the settings, lead to a better estimate of $x_{(\Gamma)}$, but the gain is often rather limited, at the expense of performing a more complex experiment.

In the classic clinical dose-finding setup, extensions of U&D have been obtained:

a) when the treatments have a factorial structure, e.g., combinations of two agents;

b) when one considers simultaneous outcomes, e.g., toxicity and efficacy of a drug;

c) with the introduction of covariates.

The problems mentioned in a) are tackled in general by assuming a parametric model at the design stage for the function $Q(x)$. Problems of type b) are usually solved by modelling the two responses separately but considering them jointly through a utility function (Ivanova, 2003b; Dragalin and Fedorov, 2006). About c), Ivanova and Wang (2006) have suggested a procedure similar to U&D for stratified populations in Phase I clinical trials. Rogatko (see for instance Babb and Rogatko (2001)) has developed a new approach for dose escalation, called *escalation with overdose control* (EWOC), which selects doses of an agent while controlling the probability of exceeding the maximum tolerated dose. The extension of EWOC to covariate utilization permits personalization of the dose level for each specific patient.

It must be stressed, however, that the papers just mentioned in general make use of a Bayesian apparatus, incorporating informative prior distributions, whereas the original idea of underlying the U&D design makes no parametric assumptions on $Q(x)$.

4

Multipurpose adaptive designs: Step-by-step procedures

4.1 Introduction

In the previous two chapters we have classified adaptive designs according to the construction methods of the randomization mechanism. We now look at the motivations, usually of an ethical nature, that lie beneath a vast class of adaptive designs. There are different ways of evaluating the usefulness of an experiment. One type of utility, the type we have been dealing with so far, is related to the information collected from the experiment, measured in terms of design optimality criteria. Another type is related to the output, for instance one might define the utility of an experiment in terms of the total expected outcome. Some experiments are multipurpose, aimed at improving the expected returns as well as gathering information for inference about the treatments.

In particular, in a clinical trial for comparing two or more treatments, the experimenter may have both goals in mind:

a) determining which, if any, is the superior treatment and how much better it is than the competitors;

b) favouring the allocation of patients to the treatment that appears to be superior as evidence about the treatment effects is gathered during the experiment.

The first is an inferential goal that reflects a possible benefit for future subjects. The second expresses an ethical responsibility to current subjects in the study. In order to achieve a) efficiently, b) may have to be sacrificed, and vice versa. This dilemma is described as "individual versus collective ethics". It is a special case of the "exploration versus exploitation", dilemma in the multi-armed bandit problem, which models an agent that simultaneously attempts to acquire new knowledge and optimize his or her decisions based on existing knowledge. Due to its generality, this problem is studied in wide variety of disciplines, such as engineering, game theory, control theory, operational research, information theory, simulation-based optimization, genetic algorithms, reinforcement learning, as well as clinical research.

In Chapter 5 we shall present global trade-off strategies for adaptive experiments which try to maximize different utilities simultaneously, while in this chapter we illustrate adaptive randomized allocation procedures devised for compromising between a) and b) on a step-by-step basis. It is worthwhile pointing out that the need for a compromise between different goals has already been encountered in Chapters 2 and 3 of this book, in the search for allocation procedures that combine optimality with randomness.

This chapter starts from the well-known Play-the-Winner design for binary response models with two treatments A and B, which has been introduced in Chapter 1: a success on a given treatment leads to assigning the same treatment to the next statistical unit, while a failure implies switching to the other treatment. The outstanding feature of the PW design is that the allocation proportion of each treatment converges to the relative risk of the other, so that in the long run the majority of subjects will receive the better treatment. It is a procedure with wide coverage all over the statistical design literature (see for instance Rosenberger and Lachin (2002)) but the allocations are not randomized, so one of the randomized versions presented in Section 4.2 might be preferable for practitioners: the Biased Coin Play-the-Winner, which combines ethics with randomization mimicking Efron's BCD, and the Randomized Play-the-Winner (Wei and Durham, 1978), i.e., an urn design in which more balls are added of the type that corresponds to the treatment that either has been successful or has not failed. This reinforces the probability of assigning the superior treatment more frequently in the future. The Drop-the-Loser (DL) design and its generalizations are similar types of urn design with an immediate utility concern: the treatment that has failed is penalized by subtracting some of the corresponding balls from the urn.

There are other possible ways for generating a step-by-step compromise between a) and b) by favouring at each step the treatment that appears to be superior. In Section 4.3 we discuss the one introduced by Atkinson and Biswas (2005a), based on a link function that transforms the treatment's superiority into the amount of skewness of its allocation probability.

A more methodological standpoint is presented in Section 4.4: when an experiment faces two purposes, a way to compromise is to allow the step-by-step allocation rule of the design to be "a compound" of the best target allocations with respect to the relative purposes. An example for binary responses is the so-called Doubly Adaptive Weighted Difference (DAWD) design of Section 4.4.1, due to Geraldes et al. (2006). It applies when we would like the design to be balanced and randomized, but also wish to favour a more ethical allocation.

In Section 4.5 we focus on a different type of urn model, the Randomly Reinforced Urn (RRU), which has the asymptotic property that the proportion of subjects assigned to the better treatment tends to one almost surely. This is a desirable ethical characteristic in clinical trials, but with some inferential drawbacks.

Section 4.6 is a reflection on the asymptotic inference made possible by the response-adaptive designs presented in Sections 4.2 and 4.5, highlighting the difference between the RRU and the others.

For clarity of presentation, in all the sections but the last one it is assumed that the number of treatments is just two, while Section 4.7 is devoted to showing how the results extend to $v > 2$ treatments.

4.2 Designs of play-the-winner and drop-the-loser type

These are designs motivated by immediate ethical considerations, without much concern for inferential advantages.

4.2.1 The Play-the-Winner design

For $v = 2$ treatments and binary responses with success probabilities p_A and p_B respectively, one of the most popular allocation rules is the so-called Play-the-Winner (PW) (Zelen, 1969). The first allocation is determined by tossing a fair coin; at each subsequent step, we assign the same treatment to the next statistical unit when a success is observed and in case of failure we switch to the other treatment.

A formal definition of this design is

$$\begin{aligned}\Pr\left(\delta_{n+1} = 1 \mid \delta^{(n)}, Y^{(n)}\right) &= \Pr\left(\delta_{n+1} = 1 \mid \delta_n, Y_n\right) \\ &= Y_n \delta_n + (1 - Y_n)(1 - \delta_n), \qquad n \geq 1.\end{aligned} \tag{4.1}$$

Clearly

$$\Pr\left(\delta_{n+1} = \delta_n \mid \delta^{(n)}, Y^{(n)}\right) = p_A \delta_n + p_B (1 - \delta_n)$$

and the Markov property

$$\Pr\left(\delta_{n+1} = 1 \mid \delta^{(n)}, Y^{(n)}\right) = \Pr\left(\delta_{n+1} = 1 \mid Y_n, \delta_n\right) \tag{4.2}$$

is satisfied by this design because of (4.1). This makes the asymptotics easier. In particular, (4.2) makes it possible to prove (see Section 1.11.2) that the allocation proportion of A converges to the relative risk of B, namely

$$\lim_{n \to \infty} \frac{N_{An}}{n} = \frac{q_B}{q_A + q_B} \quad a.s. \tag{4.3}$$

and conversely, so that in the long run the majority of subjects will receive the better treatment. As already pointed out, the asymptotic allocation proportion (4.3) is often regarded as an intuitively appealing target, but from a mathematical point of view in some circumstances it has shortcomings that will be formally discussed in Section 5.3. Clearly, convergence to (4.3) can be achieved also by any of the randomization methods described in Chapter 3.

The use of Play-the-Winner for clinical purposes is sometimes advocated as being "an optimal model that minimizes the number of failures" (Chow and Chang, 2007), however this claim is not supported by the theory. It is worth stressing that the PW strategy is a myopic one: each time, the decision is based only on the outcome of the most recent observation and in the long run it may be far from optimal.

In the same context, the "dual" target

$$\frac{p_A}{p_A + p_B} \tag{4.4}$$

may also be regarded as desirable, because it shares with (4.3) the advantage of assigning the better treatment to the majority of subjects, but does not appear to arise by a "natural" allocation method similar to the PW rule.

Another example of a desirable target with the same property as Play-the-Winner is the target proportional to the *odds* of positive response for each treatment (see Atkinson and Biswas (2014)), i.e.

$$\left(\frac{p_A q_B}{p_A q_B + p_B q_A}, \frac{p_B q_A}{p_B q_A + p_A q_B} \right), \tag{4.5}$$

which gives a higher proportion of allocations to the better treatment than PW, since when $p_A \geq p_B$

$$\frac{p_A q_B}{p_A q_B + p_B q_A} \geq \frac{q_B}{q_B + q_A},$$

and vice versa. Similarly, another possible desirable target would be the one proportional to the *odds ratio*

$$\left(\frac{p_A^2 q_B^2}{p_A^2 q_B + p_B^2 q_A^2}, \frac{p_B^2 q_A^2}{p_B^2 q_A^2 + p_A^2 q_B^2} \right)^t, \tag{4.6}$$

giving an even higher proportion of allocations to the better treatment, and so on.

4.2.2 The Biased Coin Play-the-Winner

The challenge to provide a randomized version was taken up by Wei and Durham (1978), as we shall see in Section 4.2.3. There is, moreover, a simple way of randomizing the PW design that parallels Efron's BCD and, although not popularized in the statistical literature, is at least useful as an example.

Suppose that a success on a given treatment leads to assigning the same treatment to the next patient not with certainty, but with probability $p \in [1/2; 1]$, while a failure implies switching to the other treatment, with the same probability p; we let the first allocation be to either treatment with equal probabilities. We call this design BC(p)-PW. Efron's BCD(p) (see Section 2.4.1) has allocation probability

$$\Pr\left(\delta_{n+1} = 1 \mid \delta^{(n)}\right) = \frac{1}{2} + \left(\frac{1}{2} - p\right) \operatorname{sgn}(D_n),$$

which can be seen as a weighted average of the two probabilities

$$\Pr\left(\delta_{n+1} = 1 \mid \delta^{(n)}\right) = \frac{1}{2} - \frac{1}{2}\operatorname{sgn}(D_n)$$

and

$$\Pr\left(\delta_{n+1} = 1 \mid \delta^{(n)}\right) = \frac{1}{2},$$

corresponding to the balanced deterministic design and to the Completely Randomized one, with weights $2p - 1$ and $2(1 - p)$, respectively. The BC(p)-PW rule too has an allocation probability that is a weighted average of the PW and the Completely Randomized ones , with the same weights $2p - 1$ and $2(1-p)$; for $p = 1$ we get PW, while for $p = 1/2$ it is CR, so BC(p)-PW is a combination of ethics and randomization.

The BC(p)-PW is a Markovian design, since at each step $n \geq 1$ the probability of the next allocation depends only on the most recent observation. Since

$$\Pr(Y_n = 1 \mid \delta_n) = p_A \delta_n + p_B(1-\delta_n),$$

then

$$\begin{aligned}
\Pr\left(\delta_{n+1} = \delta_n \mid \delta^{(n)}, Y^{(n)}\right) &= p \Pr(Y_n = 1 \mid \delta_n) + (1-p)\Pr(Y_n = 0 \mid \delta_n) \\
=& p\left[p_A\delta_n + p_B(1-\delta_n)\right] + (1-p)\left[q_A\delta_n + q_B(1-\delta_n)\right] \\
=& \left[pp_A + (1-p)q_A\right]\delta_n + \left[pp_B + (1-p)q_B\right](1-\delta_n) \\
=& \tilde{p}_A\delta_n + \tilde{p}_B(1-\delta_n),
\end{aligned} \tag{4.7}$$

where

$$\tilde{p}_A = pp_A + (1-p)q_A \quad \text{and} \quad \tilde{p}_B = pp_B + (1-p)q_B. \tag{4.8}$$

Definition (4.8) has the effect of "shrinking" both p_A and p_B towards the mid value $1/2$, but preserving their ranking.

The Markov property (4.7) of this randomized design is identical to a PW with success probabilities $\tilde{p}_A$ and $\tilde{p}_B$. Therefore, by exactly the same arguments as for the PW, this design will converge almost surely to the target allocation

$$\lim_{n\to\infty} \frac{N_{A,n}}{n} = \frac{\tilde{q}_B}{\tilde{q}_A + \tilde{q}_B} = \frac{(1-p)p_B + pq_B}{(1-p)(p_A+p_B) + p(q_A+q_B)}, \tag{4.9}$$

where $\tilde{q}_A = 1 - \tilde{p}_A = pq_A + (1-p)p_A$ and $\tilde{q}_B = 1 - \tilde{p}_B = pq_B + (1-p)p_B$.

Thus introducing the above biased coin randomization "dampens" the long-term effect of the PW. In the long run, a majority of units will still receive the better treatment, but in a smaller percentage as compared to the PW target, as the following numerical example shows.

Example 4.1 *Let $p_A = 0.75$ and $p_B = 0.50$, the PW asymptotic allocation proportion of treatment A is $q_B/(q_A+q_B) = 2/3$, whereas a BC-PW with $p = 3/4$, say, gives the following asymptotic target*

$$\frac{(1-p)p_B + pq_B}{(1-p)(p_A+p_B) + p(q_A+q_B)} = \frac{4}{7} < \frac{2}{3}.$$

4.2.3 Wei and Durham's Randomized Play-the-Winner

The randomized version of PW due to Wei and Durham (1978) is based on an urn mechanism. Urn models, already visited in Chapter 2 as a useful device to introduce randomness, play an important role also in the context of response-adaptive randomization, by letting the number of balls added or subtracted from the urn at each step depend on the past responses.

Suppose we have an urn with $u > 0$ balls of type A and u balls of type B. At each step a ball is drawn at random and replaced: if it is of type j ($j = A, B$), treatment j is assigned. Then the contents of the urn are updated according to the observed response: a success of treatment A or a failure of treatment B leads to placing $\beta > 0$ extra balls of type A and $\alpha > 0$ extra balls of type B into the urn; conversely, a success of treatment B or a failure of treatment A leads to the addition of β extra balls of type B and α extra balls of type A, with $\beta > \alpha \geq 0$. It is worth pointing out once more that, outside the urn metaphor, u, α and β may be just real numbers and not necessarily integers. In this way

1. each time a constant number $\alpha + \beta$ of balls is added, so that the urn is of a balanced type (see Chapter 2);
2. more balls will pile up in the urn of the type corresponding to the treatment with more successes or fewer failures.

The analogies of this procedure with mechanisms of the reinforcement learning type are evident.

The common notation for this design is RPW(u, α, β). A simplified version is with $\alpha = 0$, namely every time we just reinforce the probability of extracting the treatment that either has been successful or, alternatively, has not failed. RPW$(u, 0, \beta)$ is the version that has become most commonly known as the Randomized Play-the-Winner rule.

A formal definition of the RPW assignment rule can be given within the Generalized Pólya Urn (GPU) framework of Chapter 2:

$$\Pr\left(\delta_{n+1} = 1 \mid \delta^{(n)}, Y^{(n)}\right) = \frac{W_{An}}{W_{An} + W_{Bn}}, \qquad n \geq 1, \qquad (4.10)$$

where W_{An}, W_{Bn} denote the number of balls of type A and B, respectively, in the urn after n assignments. If $R_n(j, l)$ is the number of balls of type l that will be added into the urn given the current assignment j, then

$$\begin{aligned} R_n(j, j) &= \beta Y_n + \alpha(1 - Y_n) \qquad & j = A, B \\ R_n(j, l) &= \alpha Y_n + \beta(1 - Y_n) \qquad & j \neq l \end{aligned}$$

so that the mean reinforcement matrix, i.e., the generating matrix,

$$\mathbf{H}_n = \begin{pmatrix} \beta p_A + \alpha q_A & \alpha p_A + \beta q_A \\ \alpha p_B + \beta q_B & \beta p_B + \alpha q_B \end{pmatrix} \qquad (4.11)$$

does not depend on n, i.e., $\mathbf{H}_n = \mathbf{H}$ (namely the urn process is time-homogeneous) and it has positive entries. Thus, as shown in Chapter 2, the asymptotic results of Athreya and Karlin (1968) hold. Indeed, using the notation of (4.8), if we let $\beta/(\alpha +$

$\beta) = p$, the generating matrix $\mathbf{H}$ in (4.11) can be rewritten as

$$\mathbf{H} = (\alpha + \beta) \begin{pmatrix} \tilde{p}_A & \tilde{q}_A \\ \tilde{q}_B & \tilde{p}_B \end{pmatrix},$$

so that $\alpha + \beta$ is the maximum eigenvalue of $\mathbf{H}$, whose associated left eigenvector is

$$\left(\frac{\tilde{q}_B}{\tilde{q}_A + \tilde{q}_B}, \frac{\tilde{q}_A}{\tilde{q}_A + \tilde{q}_B} \right)^t.$$

Thus one obtains

$$\lim_{n\to\infty} \frac{N_{An}}{n} = \frac{\tilde{q}_B}{\tilde{q}_A + \tilde{q}_B} = \frac{\alpha p_B + \beta q_B}{\alpha(p_A + p_B) + \beta(q_A + q_B)} \quad \text{a.s.} \tag{4.12}$$

which is (4.9), the "shrunk" target of the BC-PW in Section 4.2.1 with $p = \beta/(\alpha+\beta)$.

It must be stressed that for the most common rule RPW$(u, 0, \beta)$ the asymptotic allocation proportion (4.12) becomes $q_B/(q_A+q_B)$, namely the RPW$(u, 0, \beta)$ design has the same asymptotic proportion of units assigned to A as the Play-the-Winner one.

Although the RPW rule is very popular in the design literature, it has some disturbing features as regards the convergence of the allocation proportion to its limit, namely the asymptotic behaviour of N_{An}/n and its speed of convergence depend in general on the values of p_A and p_B (Athreya and Karlin, 1968; Smythe, 1996). Indeed, if $p_A + p_B \leq 3/2$, the limiting distribution of the allocation proportion N_{An}/n is normal, although the order of convergence as well as the asymptotic variance change depending on whether $p_A + p_B < 3/2$ or $p_A + p_B = 3/2$; while when $p_A + p_B > 3/2$, the limiting distribution is non-normal and it strongly depends on the initial urn composition (see e.g. Rosenberger and Lachin (2002); Matthews and Rosenberger (1997)). This is a clear example in which the use of simulations based on Method ii) discussed in Section 1.14 to investigate the asymptotic properties of the design may lead to wrong conclusions. Indeed, it might be erroneous to extrapolate the asymptotic behaviour of this design from simulations based on the estimated values of p_A and p_B alone, since the very convergence depends on the true treatment effects.

One may also wonder about comparing RPW(u, α, β) and BC$(\beta/(\alpha + \beta))$-PW, since they share the same limiting allocation (4.12). There is a remarkable difference from the viewpoint of the design process $\{\delta_n\}_{n\in\mathbb{N}}$. In the BC-PW, $\{\delta_n\}_{n\in\mathbb{N}}$ is Markovian; at each step only the most recent allocation and response matter, whereas for the RPW(u, α, β) the urn composition is determined step-by-step by the entire past history of the experiment.

4.2.4 Drop-the-Loser and Generalized Drop-the-Loser

Another important randomized rule based on a similar idea is the so-called Drop-the Loser. In general, a "drop-the-loser" design is one that permits dropping the inferior treatment arms. Typically, this procedure is performed in two stages: at the end of the first stage the arm or arms deemed to be inferior will be dropped, based on some pre-specified criterion; then the winners will proceed to the next stage. These designs are also called "Pick-the-winner" (Simon and Simon, 2013). Not much in-depth analysis of them exists so far, so in this book we focus instead on a modified version, also called "Drop-the-Loser", suggested by Ivanova et al. (2000), see also Ivanova and Flournoy (2001) and Ivanova (2003a), particularly attractive due to its small variability.

Ivanova's Drop-the-Loser (DL) is an urn design for binary response models where the probability of assigning a treatment decreases when the treatment fails. In the DL rule, instead of adding balls to the urn to reward successful treatments, balls are removed when failures are observed. Clearly this might lead to the extinction of a type of ball after a while, namely dropping a treatment arm forever, which is not the intention of this design. Thus a refurbishment mechanism is also introduced.

More precisely, consider an urn containing three types of balls: balls of types A and B representing the two treatments and balls of type O, called *immigration balls*. We start with w_O, w_A and w_B balls of type O, A and B, respectively. At each step, a ball is drawn at random. If a ball of type A or B is selected, the corresponding treatment is assigned and the response is observed. If the treatment is a failure, the ball is not replaced. If it is a success, the ball is replaced and consequently the urn composition remains unchanged. If an immigration ball (type O) is selected, no subject is treated, and the ball is returned to the urn together with two additional treatment balls, one of each treatment type. This procedure is repeated until a treatment ball is drawn and the subject treated accordingly. No immigration ball is ever added to the urn. With this type of design, care should be exerted in defining what is meant by *stage* k of the experiment, as the number of steps no longer corresponds to the number of treatment allocations, but only to the number of times balls are extracted. In other words, if $\tilde{N}_{jm}$ is the number of allocations of treatment j ($j = A, B$) up to the first m extractions, it is no longer true that $\tilde{N}_{Am} + \tilde{N}_{Bm} = m$, since the number of treated subjects is $\leq m$.

The DL is evidently an adaptive randomized design. The following asymptotic result is proved by Ivanova (2003a):

$$\lim_{m\to\infty} \frac{\tilde{N}_{Am}}{\tilde{N}_{Am} + \tilde{N}_{Bm}} = \frac{q_B}{q_A + q_B} \qquad \text{in probability,} \tag{4.13}$$

which is similar, but not equivalent, to (4.3). Furthermore, Ivanova (2003a) shows that

$$\sqrt{\tilde{N}_{Am} + \tilde{N}_{Bm}} \left(\frac{\tilde{N}_{Am}}{\tilde{N}_{Am} + \tilde{N}_{Bm}} - \frac{q_B}{q_A + q_B} \right) \to^d N(0; \sigma^2_{DL}), \tag{4.14}$$

with

$$\sigma^2_{DL} = \frac{q_A q_B (p_A + p_B)}{(q_A + q_B)^3}.$$

We point out that the convergence in (4.14) has a different interpretation with respect to the asymptotic normality of the allocation proportion discussed in Chapter 3. Indeed, let τ_n be the number of balls that are extracted in order to allocate the first n subjects to the treatments, then $\tau_n = n + \sum_{i=1}^{n} O_i$, where O_i denotes the number of immigration balls that have been drawn for allocating the ith statistical unit, so that $N_{An} = \tilde{N}_{A\tau_n}$, but the random nature of τ_n is not taken into account by (4.14).

Sun et al. (2007) have suggested the following extension of the DL rule, called Generalized Drop-the-Loser, also providing a general asymptotic framework by which it is possible to derive the almost sure convergence of the allocation proportion to the target and its asymptotic normality (instead of (4.13) and (4.14) as shown below).

Suppose that the balls are the same as above, namely two types corresponding to the treatments and one to immigration. When an immigration ball (type O) is drawn, no treatment is assigned and the ball is returned to the urn along with $a_j > 0$ type j treatment balls ($j = A, B$); a_j is not necessarily an integer. This step is repeated until a treatment ball is drawn. When a treatment ball is drawn, the unit is assigned to that treatment. Let Y_n be the observed outcome of the nth unit that is assigned to treatment j. Then a random number $R_n(j;j)$ of balls of type j are added to the urn, with $R_n(j;j)$ an increasing function of Y_n.

For $a_A = a_B = 1$ and $R_n(j;j) = 0$ or -1, according to whether we observe success or failure, we get DL as a special case.

If the urn process is time-homogeneous (i.e., $E[R_n(j;j)]$ does not depend on n) with $-1 < E[R_n(j;j)] < 0$, the authors prove that

$$\lim_{n\to\infty} \frac{N_{An}}{n} = \frac{a_A/q_A}{a_A/q_A + a_B/q_B}, \qquad \text{a.s.} \tag{4.15}$$

and furthermore

$$\sqrt{n}\left(\frac{N_{An}}{n} - \frac{a_A/q_A}{a_A/q_A + a_B/q_B}\right) \to^d N(0; \sigma^2_{GDL}), \tag{4.16}$$

where

$$\sigma^2_{GDL} = \frac{a_A a_B q_A q_B \left(a_B p_A + a_A p_B\right)}{\left(a_B q_A + a_A q_B\right)^3}.$$

Thus, σ^2_{GDL} (and therefore σ^2_{DL}) is a measure of the design variability and, from Chapter 3, it follows that the GDL attains the lower bound for the asymptotic variance (3.4) of a design targeting

$$\frac{\frac{a_A}{q_A}}{\frac{a_A}{q_A} + \frac{a_B}{q_B}}.$$

To avoid possible confusion, we stress that this lower bound refers to an asymptotically normal design converging to the given target (see Section 3.3).

Hu and Rosenberger (2006) have made a comparative study of the RPW and the DL rules for different values of p_A and p_B based on simulations with $n = 100$ and $n = 1000$ (see Tables 8.1 and 8.2 of Hu and Rosenberger (2006)). By comparing the asymptotic and simulated means of $n^{-1}N_{in}$ and the asymptotic and simulated variances of $n^{-1/2}N_{in}$, their study yields results favouring the adoption of the DL rule.

The DL design is much praised in the literature (for instance in Hu and Rosenberger (2006)) for its small variability, which implies higher statistical power for statistical treatment comparison.

Suitable choices of a_A and a_B would make it possible to converge to any given target proportion. However, in that case a_A and a_B might depend on the unknown parameters, i.e., $a_j = a_j(p_A, p_B)$ $(j = A, B)$, and thus would have to be estimated each time by $\hat{a}_{jn} = a_j(\hat{p}_{An}, \hat{p}_{Bn})$. In this case, suitable assumptions on the rate of convergence of $\hat{a}_{jn} \to a_j$ guarantee that (4.15) and (4.16) continue to hold.

Delayed responses may be allowed for by delaying the possible addition of balls to the urn until the subject's response is observed, while continuing to extract from the urn (Zhang et al., 2007a).

4.2.5 Further extensions of the PW design

Several other randomized extensions of PW have been suggested in the literature, like the success-driven designs to be discussed in Section 4.5, where balls of the same type are added in case of success and failures are ignored, and the Failure-Driven Designs (FDD) where β balls of the opposite type are added in case of failure. A description of the latter, as well as several numerical comparisons with the classical RPW and with DL, can be found in Atkinson and Biswas (2014), without formal properties. It is easy to see that the mean reinforcement matrix of the FDD is

$$\mathbf{H}_n = \begin{pmatrix} 0 & \beta q_A \\ \beta q_B & 0 \end{pmatrix} \tag{4.17}$$

which does not depend on n. By a similar argument to Section 4.2.3 one obtains

$$\lim_{n\to\infty} \frac{N_{An}}{n} = \frac{\sqrt{q_B}}{\sqrt{q_A} + \sqrt{q_B}} \quad \text{a.s.} \tag{4.18}$$

This target is $\geq 1/2$ when $p_A \geq p_B$ but is always less than the PW target in (4.3). In Atkinson and Biswas (2014) it is repeatedly stated that simulations of the Failure-Driven Design show it to be less variable than DL, but the comparison is between designs with different targets.

The Birth-and-Death urn design (Ivanova et al., 2000) is a more general version of Drop-the-Loser. When a treatment is successful, one ball of the same type is added to the urn. In case of failure, one ball of the same type is taken out from the urn. Since certain treatments can "die out" a Poisson immigration process to replenish the urn is introduced. The Maximum Likelihood estimators of the success probabilities are obtained, their consistency is proved and their limiting distributions is obtained using martingale theory. The authors prove that the treatment allocation of A may converge either to 0, or to a random quantity, or to

$$\frac{\frac{1}{(q_A - p_A)}}{\frac{1}{(q_A - p_A)} + \frac{1}{(q_B - p_B)}},$$

if $p_A < 1/2$ and $p_B < 1/2$.

In conclusion, it is not clear wether these proposals are a substantial improvement over the previously mentioned designs.

4.3 Bandyopadhyay and Biswas' link-based design

In order to favour step-by-step the assignment of the treatment that appears to be superior, Bandyopadhyay and Biswas (2001) have introduced a design for normal homoscedastic response trials (1.8) based on a function that links the difference between the treatment effects to the ethical skewness of the allocation probability. Let $J(\cdot)$ denote the cdf of a random variable that is symmetric around 0; the authors suggest to set

$$\Pr\left(\delta_{n+1} = 1 \mid \delta^{(n)}, Y^{(n)}\right) = J\left(\hat{\mu}_A - \hat{\mu}_B\right), \tag{4.19}$$

so that if $\hat{\mu}_A > \hat{\mu}_B$ then the probability of allocating treatment A to the next statistical unit is greater than 1/2.

In practice, the role of $J(\cdot)$ is to transform the treatment differences into suitably chosen ethical targets and a very natural choice consists in assuming J as the cumulative distribution function (cdf) of a normal random variable $N(0; T^2)$, namely setting $J(x) = \Phi(x/T)$, where the non-negative parameter T controls the degree of skewness of the assignments. Under this choice the design (4.19) becomes

$$\Pr\left(\delta_{n+1} = 1 \mid \delta^{(n)}, Y^{(n)}\right) = \Phi\left(\frac{\hat{\mu}_A - \hat{\mu}_B}{T}\right). \tag{4.20}$$

As T increases the allocations tend to be randomized like an unbiased coin. This design is called *link-based* or BB, from the initials of the authors. The authors prove that, as n tends to infinity,

$$\lim_{n\to\infty} \frac{N_{An}}{n} = \Phi\left(\frac{\mu_A - \mu_B}{T}\right) \quad a.s. \tag{4.21}$$

and thus, from an asymptotic point of view,

- the majority of the subjects will be assigned to the better treatment,
- the ethical gain in favouring the better treatment corresponds exactly to the step-by-step bias towards the treatment that appears to be superior.

If the responses are normal homoscedastic with standard deviation σ, the choice $T = \sqrt{2}\sigma$ gives

$$\Pr\left(\delta_{n+1} = 1 \mid \delta^{(n)}, Y^{(n)}\right) \to \Pr(Y_A > Y_B)$$

as n goes to infinity. Some numerical calculations and simulations of the properties of this design can be found in Atkinson and Biswas (2014).

As discussed by Bandyopadhyay and Biswas (2001), a critical concern is the choice of T, which is strictly related to both the magnitude of the treatment effects and the importance of ethical aspects in the trial. For instance:

- when $\mu_A - \mu_B = 0.5$, the choice $T = 0.3$ gives an asymptotic allocation proportion to A around 95%,
- for a difference between the treatment effects equal to 1, if $T = 1$ then $\lim_{n\to\infty} \pi_n = 0.84$.

Thus any choice of T could induce strongly unbalanced groups, which may be desirable from an ethical point of view but could be negative for inference. Indeed, as shown in Chapter 2, large departures from balance could induce a significant loss of precision in terms of both i) power of the test and ii) variance of the estimated treatment difference.

A proper choice of T can be made only if we have some a priori information about the true values of the treatment effects, scaled with respect to the variances of the treatment responses. Otherwise, T could itself be a function of the unknown treatment effects: this possibility remains to be investigated.

4.4 The compound probability approach

Obtaining a design (i.e., an allocation rule) by the combination of two separate allocation rules, one for each of two different purposes, is what we call the *compound probability* approach. For instance, one of the two allocation probabilities that are combined may reflect efficient inference (design optimality) and the other an ethical concern. When the concern is threefold, for instance when it involves randomness, optimality and ethics, a more sophisticated approach is required, possibly combining allocation probabilities that are already combinations of allocations.

A combination of allocation probabilities can be achieved by means of any increasing transformation $\varphi : [0,1]^2 \to [0,1]$ such that

$$\varphi(x; y) = 1 - \varphi(1-x; 1-y), \qquad \forall\, x, y \in (0,1)^2 \tag{4.22}$$

(i.e., the same as Condition C0) of Section 3.4 in Chapter 3), so that the compound probabilities of assigning A and B still add up to 1.

There are several ways of achieving a compound probability. Taking a weighted average with weights whose sum is 1 is the simplest, as in the case of the BC-PW, in which this method is used to combine ethics with randomness. Another intuitive example is taking the product of the odds of the original allocation probabilities as the new odds of allocating A and B.

Example 4.2 *Combining the PW target $q_B/(q_A + q_B)$ with the dual ethical target $p_A/(p_A+p_B)$ by means of this method of the odds, the result is the odds-based target mentioned in Section 4.2.1, namely $p_Aq_B/(p_Bq_A + p_Aq_B)$.*

Both the weighted average and the odds method have the symmetry property (4.22), but other types of mathematical mean (e.g., geometric mean, harmonic mean, power mean) do not, so care is needed in the definition.

4.4.1 The Doubly Adaptive Weighted Difference design

The Doubly Adaptive Weighted Difference (DAWD) design by Geraldes et al. (2006) is a compromise design for binary responses that applies when ideally we would seek an almost balanced randomized design, but also wish to favour a more ethical allocation of patients. At each step the probability of the next assignment is a compromise between one component devised to mitigate imbalance and another devised to skew the allocations towards the better treatment in a way that takes into account the difference in treatment effects, similarly to the skewed design of Section 4.3.

Let $g(\cdot)$ and $h(\cdot)$ be two real continuous functions with range in $[0, 1]$, both standing for the probability of assigning treatment A at the next step; $g(\cdot)$ is dictated by ethics, and is an increasing function of the estimated difference at step k of the success probabilities p_A, p_B, with $g(0) = 1/2$; $h(\cdot)$ is dictated by balance and is a decreasing function of the relative imbalance between A and B, with $h(0) = 1/2$. Symmetry between the two treatments is preserved by taking

$$\begin{aligned} g(-x) &= 1 - g(x) \qquad \text{for all } x \in [-1, 1] \\ h(-x) &= 1 - h(x) \qquad \text{for all } x \in [-1, 1]. \end{aligned}$$

The two functions $g(\cdot)$ and $h(\cdot)$ are then combined by weights $\omega \in [0; 1)$ and $1 - \omega$, that reflect the relative importance of ethics and inference, respectively, to get the following allocation rule:

$$\Pr\left(\delta_{n+1} = 1 \mid \delta^{(n)}, Y^{(n)}\right) = \omega g(\hat{p}_{An} - \hat{p}_{Bn}) + (1 - \omega) h\left(2\pi_n - 1\right), \quad n \geq 2n_0 \tag{4.23}$$

where n_0 is the number of subjects assigned to either treatment in the initial pilot study performed to derive non-trivial estimates of the success probabilities p_A and p_B.

By the continuity of $g(\cdot)$ and $h(\cdot)$, it can be proved that the asymptotic allocation proportion to A of the DAWD design is the unique solution π^*_{dawd} in $(0, 1)$ of the equation:

$$\pi = \omega g(p_A - p_B) + (1 - \omega) h\left(2\pi - 1\right). \tag{4.24}$$

Without any ethics or cost constraint, namely for $\omega = 0$, this design is the same as Wei's Biased Coin Design defined in Chapter 2, since at each step n $h(\cdot)$ is a function of the relative imbalance $n^{-1}D_n = 2\pi_n - 1$. Thus any of the allocation probabilities $f(x)$ mentioned in Section 2.4.3 are candidates for h. As regards the function $g(\cdot)$, an extreme choice is given by $g(x) = 1$ if $x > 0$, $g(x) = 0$ if $x < 0$, which corresponds to the rationale of the PW design, where we "estimate" $p_A - p_B > 0$ when A is successful or B fails and < 0 when B is successful or A fails. Otherwise, in the same spirit as the link-based design (Bandyopadhyay and Biswas, 2002) discussed in Section 4.3, we could assume a link function $J : [-1; 1] \rightarrow [0; 1]$ that translates the current superiority of a given treatment into a suitable skewness in its favour. We have ruled out the possibility $\omega = 1$, but it is true to say that as $\omega \to 1$, the allocation is based almost entirely on the estimated difference between the success probabilities, obtaining in this way an analogue for binary responses of the skewed design of Bandyopadhyay and Biswas (2002) for normal ones.

There is very little discussion in Geraldes et al. (2006) about the choice of the weights ω and $1-\omega$. We postpone any considerations on this choice to Chapter 5.

Example 4.3 *If we take the functions $g(\cdot)$ and $h(\cdot)$ to be linear by letting*

$$h(x) = \frac{1-x}{2} \qquad \textit{and} \qquad g(x) = \frac{1+x}{2},$$

then from (4.24) there follows that

$$\lim_{n\to\infty} \frac{N_{An}}{n} = \frac{1}{2} + \frac{\omega}{2-\omega}\frac{(p_A - p_B)}{2}.$$

In particular, for $\omega = 1/2$, the asymptotic allocation proportion of treatment A is

$$\pi^*_{dawd} = \frac{1}{2} + \frac{p_A - p_B}{6}.$$

4.4.2 Atkinson and Biswas' skewed D_A-optimum Biased Coin Design

Another design obtained through the same compound probability approach is the skewed D_A-optimum Biased Coin Design for the homoscedastic normal model given by Atkinson and Biswas (2005b). This is a compromise between minimizing at each step the variance of the estimated treatment difference, while at the same time preserving a suitable degree of randomness, and favouring the allocations to the better treatment. The idea of Atkinson and Biswas (2005b) is to combine the randomized allocation rule of the D_A-optimum Biased Coin Design modified according to the suggestion of Ball et al. (1993) (see Section 2.6), with (4.20), the ethically skewed rule of Bandyopadhyay and Biswas (2001).

The allocation-adaptive design of Ball et al. (1993) assigns treatment A to the $(n+1)$st unit with probability

$$\Pr\left(\delta_{n+1} = 1 \mid \delta^{(n)}\right) = \frac{\left(1 + \frac{N_{Bn}}{nN_{An}}\right)^{\frac{1}{\zeta}}}{\left(1 + \frac{N_{Bn}}{nN_{An}}\right)^{\frac{1}{\zeta}} + \left(1 + \frac{N_{An}}{nN_{Bn}}\right)^{\frac{1}{\zeta}}}, \qquad (4.25)$$

where ζ is a non-negative parameter that controls randomization, and Atkinson and Biswas (2005b) obtain the following allocation probability:

$$\Pr\left(\delta_{n+1} = 1 \mid \delta^{(n)}, Y^{(n)}\right) = \frac{\Phi\left(\frac{\hat\theta_A - \hat\theta_B}{T}\right)\left(1 + \frac{N_{Bn}}{nN_{An}}\right)^{\frac{1}{\zeta}}}{\Phi\left(\frac{\hat\theta_A - \hat\theta_B}{T}\right)\left(1 + \frac{N_{Bn}}{nN_{An}}\right)^{\frac{1}{\zeta}} + \Phi\left(\frac{\hat\theta_B - \hat\theta_A}{T}\right)\left(1 + \frac{N_{An}}{nN_{Bn}}\right)^{\frac{1}{\zeta}}}.$$

This type of compound probability corresponds to taking the product of the odds of the original allocations as the new odds of allocating A and B. The convergence of the allocations proportion of A is to the target

$$\Phi\left(\frac{\theta_A - \theta_B}{T}\right).$$

The properties of this design have been investigated by the authors mainly by means of numerical studies.

4.5 Randomly Reinforced Urn designs

So far, the designs of this chapter are for binary or normal responses and share the property that the allocation proportion converges to a target which is strictly between 0 and 1 for all the treatments. There is a different type of randomized adaptive design obtained by means of an urn model, the so-called *Randomly Reinforced Urn* (RRU) in which the proportion of patients allocated to the better treatment in the long run will approach 1 almost surely. RRU designs for experiments with binary outcomes were introduced by Durham and Yu (1990) as a modification of the Randomized Play-the-Winner (RPW) scheme. One major feature of the RRUs is to be *success-driven*, namely to reward only successful treatments, in other words balls are not added to the urn if the treatment is a failure. The designs have been extended to experiments with continuous responses by Beggs (2005) and Muliere et al. (2006b). A very clear overview is given by Flournoy et al. (2012), and we follow their presentation.

Let the statistical model for the response be a member of the exponential family, as in Chapter 1. We introduce a real non-negative measurable bounded function $\mathcal{H}(y)$ on the range of the outcomes, which quantifies a reward obtained from the response y.

Example 4.4 *For binary outcomes, the reward could also be* 0 *for failure or* 1 *for success, so that* $\mathcal{H}(y) = y$. *More generally,* $\mathcal{H}$ *can be the identity function when the distributions of* Y *conditional on the treatments are non-negative and have bounded support. In typical applications with normal responses,* $\mathcal{H}(\cdot)$ *will be taken to be a monotonic function.*

To define RRU, consider an urn initially containing $w_A > 0$ balls of type A and $w_B > 0$ balls of type B. At each step k, the extracted ball is replaced in the urn together with $\mathcal{H}(Y_k)$ additional balls of the same type. After n steps, the probability of assigning each treatment is proportional to the number of balls of that type in the urn, namely

$$W_{An} = w_A + \sum_{k=1}^{n} \delta_k \mathcal{H}(Y_k),$$
$$W_{Bn} = w_B + \sum_{k=1}^{n} (1 - \delta_k) \mathcal{H}(Y_k).$$

The quantities W_{An} and W_{Bn} stand for the cumulated observed responses (transformed by $\mathcal{H}$) to treatments A and B respectively, augmented by the initial number of balls of that type in the urn.

Let m_A and m_B be the expected urn reinforcements, i.e.,

$$m_A = \int \mathcal{H}(y) \mathcal{L}_A(dy) \qquad \text{and} \qquad m_B = \int \mathcal{H}(y) \mathcal{L}_B(dy),$$

where $\mathcal{L}_A$ and $\mathcal{L}_B$ are the distributions of the outcomes under treatment A and B respectively. A fundamental result proved by Li et al. (1997) for dichotomous responses and extended to general responses by Beggs (2005), Muliere et al. (2006b) and Aletti et al. (2009) is

$$\text{if} \quad m_A > m_B, \quad \text{then} \quad \lim_{n \to \infty} \frac{W_{An}}{W_{An} + W_{Bn}} = 1 \quad \text{a.s.}$$

Not surprisingly, the proportion of subjects allocated to A and B has the same limit as the urn composition (see May and Flournoy (2009)), namely

$$\text{if} \quad m_A > m_B, \quad \text{then} \quad \lim_{n \to \infty} \frac{N_{An}}{n} = 1 \quad \text{a.s.}$$

Furthermore, if $m_A > m_B$ then there exists a random variable η, almost certainly finite, such that

$$\lim_{n \to \infty} \frac{N_{Bn}}{n^{m_B/m_A}} = \eta^2 \qquad a.s. \tag{4.26}$$

To apply this in clinical trials, suppose that conditionally on treatment A the responses have mean μ_A and on treatment B have mean μ_B, and suppose that A is preferred to B if $\mu_A > \mu_B$. If we choose a function $\mathcal{H}(\cdot)$ such that $m_A > m_B$ if and only if $\mu_A > \mu_B$ and $m_A = m_B$ if and only if $\mu_A = \mu_B$, then the RRU design allocates subjects to the superior treatment with probability converging to one as n goes to infinity. Hence these designs are asymptotically very desirable from an ethical point of view. However, for any given sample size RRU tends to generate strongly unbalanced groups and the inferential procedures for comparing treatment effects based on these designs are usually characterized by very low power . Besides, from an asymptotic viewpoint, there is a clash with the requirement of randomness in the allocation process, which limits its applicability in practice. For these reasons, the reinforcement scheme of the urn has been modified by Aletti et al. (2013) to construct a design that asymptotically targets an allocation proportion ρ very near the optimal ethical target but lying in $(0,1)$, and this urn model has been called the Modified Randomly Reinforced Urn.

Simulations carried out for binary and normal responses show that the convergence of the RRU design to the optimal ethical target is typically slow and in finite samples the variability of the number of patients allocated to the superior treatment is high. It is clear that different choices of the function $\mathcal{H}(\cdot)$ lead to different properties for the RRU design, in terms of the distributions of allocations and rate of convergence.

When the two treatments are equivalent, that is $\mu_A = \mu_B$, then $m_A = m_B$ and the sequence

$$\left\{ Z_n = \frac{W_{An}}{W_{An} + W_{Bn}} \right\}_{n\in\mathbb{N}}$$

converges almost surely to a random limit Z_∞ in $[0,1]$ (Muliere et al., 2006a), whose distribution is generally unknown; this (random) limit proportion is not concentrated in any point mass and

$$\lim_{n\to\infty} \frac{N_{An}}{n} = Z_\infty \quad a.s.$$

4.6 Asymptotic inference for multipurpose designs

For all the designs discussed in this chapter, apart from RRU, the proportion of allocations to treatment A converges to a quantity strictly between 0 and 1, so that the statements of Theorem 1.3 hold true. The strong consistency and asymptotic normality of the MLEs of the parameters of interest is established.

For the DAWD, Geraldes et al. (2006) also show that estimators of p_A and p_B which are "sufficiently close" to the MLEs, namely the sample proportions, like the "Bayesian" estimators

$$\hat{p}_{An} = \frac{\sum_{k=1}^n \delta_k Y_k + 1}{N_{An} + 2} \qquad \text{and} \qquad \hat{p}_{Bn} = \frac{\sum_{k=1}^n (1-\delta_k) Y_k + 1}{N_{Bn} + 2},$$

or the Wilson estimators

$$\hat{p}_{An} = \frac{\sum_{k=1}^n \delta_k Y_k + 2}{N_{An} + 4} \qquad \text{and} \qquad \hat{p}_{Bn} = \frac{\sum_{k=1}^n (1-\delta_k) Y_k + 2}{N_{Bn} + 4},$$

are strongly consistent and asymptotically normal.

For RRU designs, when $m_A \neq m_B$, the allocation proportion to treatment A converges to 0 or 1 so that Theorem 1.3 cannot be applied. Notwithstanding the fact that in an RRU design the conditional probability of allocating the nth subject to the inferior treatment converges to zero, the random numbers of subjects N_{An} and N_{Bn} both converge to infinity almost surely, as the total number n of subjects goes to infinity. This result, proved in May and Flournoy (2009), permits the development of asymptotic inference for RRU designs. Consider the estimation of the means

(μ_A, μ_B) and the variances (σ_A^2, σ_B^2) of the responses to the treatments. May and Flournoy (2009) have considered the following estimators:

$$\hat{\mu}_{An} = \frac{\sum_{k=1}^{n} \delta_k Y_k}{N_{An}} \quad \text{and} \quad \hat{\mu}_{Bn} = \frac{\sum_{k=1}^{n}(1-\delta_k) Y_k}{N_{Bn}},$$

and

$$\hat{\sigma}_{An}^2 = \frac{\sum_{k=1}^{n} \delta_k (Y_k - \hat{\mu}_{An})^2}{N_{An}} \quad \text{and} \quad \hat{\sigma}_{Bn}^2 = \frac{\sum_{k=1}^{n}(1-\delta_k)(Y_k - \hat{\mu}_{Bn})^2}{N_{Bn}}$$

and proved that they are strongly consistent for (μ_A, μ_B) and (σ_A^2, σ_B^2) respectively. They have also proved that, both when $\mu_A = \mu_B$ and when $\mu_A \neq \mu_B$, as $n \to \infty$

$$\left(\frac{\sqrt{N_{An}}}{\sigma_A}(\hat{\mu}_{An} - \mu_A), \frac{\sqrt{N_{Bn}}}{\sigma_B}(\hat{\mu}_{Bn} - \mu_B) \right)^t \to^d N(0, \mathbf{I}_2).$$

To test

$$H_0 : \mu_A = \mu_B \qquad \text{versus} \qquad H_1 : \mu_A > \mu_B$$

a possible test statistic is

$$\zeta_n = \frac{\hat{\mu}_{An} - \hat{\mu}_{Bn}}{\sqrt{\frac{\hat{\sigma}_{An}^2}{N_{An}} + \frac{\hat{\sigma}_{Bn}^2}{N_{Bn}}}},$$

which under H_0 is asymptotically normal. When the alternative hypothesis is true, the distribution of the test statistic ζ_n is a mixture of normal distributions, namely the conditional distribution of ζ_n given the random variable η defined in (4.26) is asymptotically normal with

$$N\left(\eta \sqrt{n^{m_B/m_A}} \left(\frac{\mu_A - \mu_B}{\sigma_A} \right); 1 \right).$$

4.7 Extensions of the step-by-step strategies to the case of several treatments

Most of the designs presented so far in this chapter have a counterpart for $v > 2$ treatments. Either all the treatments are equivalent, or some of them – typically just one – will be the best. Favouring the allocation to the treatment or treatments that appear to be superior during the experiment while gathering information about all the effects is a desirable goal in this case too. Nothing very much changes for estimation of the parameters, but with more than two treatments, there is now a large number of hypotheses that one may want to test, concerning equalities versus inequalities among the treatment effects, or among a control treatment and all the other ones. Typically, these will involve contrasts among the parameters, i.e., they correspond to testing whether a linear transformation of the parameters is equal to 0 or different, or whether it is equal to 0 or greater.

For binary responses let the treatments be T_j ($j = 1, \ldots, v$) with probabilities of success $0 < p_j < 1$. Wei (1979) has extended the Play-the-Winner rule to this case introducing the Cyclic Play-the-Winner. The v treatments are ordered in a cyclic way: after each success we treat the next unit in the same way, after each failure we switch to the next treatment. This is still a Markovian design, with convergence

$$\lim_{n\to\infty} \frac{N_{jn}}{n} = \frac{1/q_j}{\sum_{k=1}^{v} (1/q_k)} \qquad a.s. \quad \forall j = 1, \ldots, v. \tag{4.27}$$

In all the urn-based designs, the definition of the allocation rule extended to $v > 2$ treatments (see also Chapter 2) clearly is

$$\Pr\left(\delta_{j,n+1} = 1 \mid \delta^{(n)}, Y^{(n)}\right) = \frac{W_{jn}}{W_{1n} + \ldots + W_{vn}}, \qquad n \geq 1,$$

for $j = 1, \ldots, v$. The addition rule is now expressed by a $v \times v$-dim matrix

$$\mathbf{R}_n = \left(R_n(j,l)\right)_{j,l=1,\ldots,v},$$

specifying the number of balls of type l that will be added into the urn given the current assignment on treatment j. For the RPW, Wei (1979)'s definition is adding $v - 1$ balls of the same type when the treatment is successful and one ball for each of the other types when it is a failure. In this case the convergence of the treatment allocation proportions is to the same target (4.27). For DL and GDL, the extension of the definition is straightforward and the convergence result is

$$\lim_{n\to\infty} \frac{N_{jn}}{n} = \frac{a_j/q_j}{a_1/q_1 + \ldots + a_v/q_v}, \qquad a.s. \quad \forall j = 1, \ldots, v. \tag{4.28}$$

Link function-based adaptive designs have been extended to more than two treatments by allocations proportional to

$$\Phi\left(\frac{\hat{\mu}_j - v^{-1}\sum_{s=1}^{v} \hat{\mu}_s}{T}\right)$$

(Atkinson and Biswas, 2014). To obtain skewed allocations combined with efficient parameter estimation for several treatments, Atkinson et al. (2011) introduce a vector $\boldsymbol{\pi}^* = (\pi_1^*, \pi_2^*, \ldots, \pi_v^*)^t$, where $\pi_1^* \geq \pi_2^* \geq \ldots \geq \pi_v^*$. They define $r(j)$ to be the rank of treatment effect j ($j = 1, \ldots, v$). Clearly the ranking of the treatments is unknown and has to be estimated at each step n by $\hat{r}_n(j)$. The definition of the design is then

$$\Pr\left(\delta_{j,n+1} = 1 \mid \delta^{(n)}, Y^{(n)}\right) = \frac{[1 + d(j,n)]^{\frac{1}{v}}\, \pi^*_{\hat{r}_n(j)}}{\sum_{j=1}^{v} [1 + d(j,n)]^{\frac{1}{v}}\, \pi^*_{\hat{r}_n(j)}}, \tag{4.29}$$

with the same meaning of $d_A(j,n)$ as in Chapter 2. Noticeably, this is not an extension of the skewed D_A-optimum Biased Coin Design discussed in Section 4.4.2, because (4.29) takes into account only the ranking of the treatments, but not how much they differ. Under "mild conditions" the authors show the convergence of the treatment allocations to the target $\left(\pi^*_{r(1)}, \pi^*_{r(2)}, \ldots, \pi^*_{r(v)}\right)$.

The extension of the definition of the RRU-design to $v \geq 2$ treatments is straightforward. For dichotomous responses Li et al. (1997) have shown that, when there is a treatment j with a unique maximum probability of success, the proportion of allocations to that treatment converges to 1 in probability. The results by Muliere et al. (2006a) for RRU designs also work for $v \geq 2$ treatments: they prove that whenever the response distribution associated to one particular treatment dominates the response distributions of the other treatments, the probability of assigning the superior treatment converges to 1.

5

Multipurpose adaptive designs: Constrained and combined optimality

5.1 Introduction

This chapter discusses methods for finding target allocations of the treatments (either as finite sample allocations, or as asymptotic proportions to be approximated in a large sample setup) that achieve a good trade-off between different experimental goals. This is different from Chapters 2 and 4, in which at each step the allocation probability is the result of a compromise between inferential optimality and randomness and/or ethical demands.

In this chapter we start from design criteria that formalize the experimental objectives and find targets that are optimal with respect to some compromise of the criteria. Within this context, two different approaches are possible (see Cook and Wong (1994)):

- constrained optimization: the target is derived by optimizing a given criterion under suitable constraints on the other criteria;
- combined optimization: the target optimizes a suitably chosen compound criterion that combines the different experimental goals by means of suitable weights.

In general the optimal target allocations derived through these approaches depend on the unknown model parameters and therefore suitable response-adaptive procedures (such as those described in Chapter 3) must be called for in order to converge to them.

After recalling a few facts about the classical optimality criteria in Section 5.2, in Section 5.3 we introduce the concept of admissibility of a target, by which we mean a target allocation that cannot be improved simultaneously with respect to all the criteria. We apply this idea to the two-treatment case when there are two design measures of loss, one is inferential and the other is the percentage of units receiving the worse treatment. Within this framework, we revisit some classical designs of the literature and introduce new ones.

Sections 5.4 and 5.5 deal with the two major approaches aimed at combining different experimental goals, namely *constrained optimization* and *combined optimization*. Either method can be applied in order to obtain "optimal" compromise targets that are also admissible with respect to the chosen pair of criteria. The equivalence of the two methods is hinted at in Section 5.5.3.

To avoid cumbersome notation, for most of the chapter we restrict ourselves to the case of just two treatments; the extension to several treatments is discussed in Section 5.6.

We stress once again that, even if the main emphasis is on clinical trials, which are special due to specific ethical concerns, the proposed methodology applies in a more general context, e.g., under economic constraints (see for instance Elfving (1952)).

5.2 Optimality of target allocations for two treatments

5.2.1 Inferentially optimal targets

Let A and B be the two treatments and suppose that the responses belong to the exponential family (1.4) parameterized as in (1.17), namely assuming that

$$\theta_A = E[Y_i \mid \delta_i = 1] \quad \text{and} \quad \theta_B = E[Y_i \mid \delta_i = 0]$$

are the treatment effects. We recall the expression of the normalized information

$$\mathbf{M}(\theta_A; \theta_B \mid \pi_n) = \text{diag}\left(\frac{\pi_n}{Var[Y_A]}; \frac{1-\pi_n}{Var[Y_B]}\right); \tag{5.1}$$

the optimal inferential target with respect to an inferential criterion Φ is the allocation

$$\pi_{\mathcal{I}}^* = \arg\min_{\pi\in[0;1]} \Phi\left[\mathbf{M}^{-1}(\theta_A; \theta_B \mid \pi)\right]. \tag{5.2}$$

The inferentially optimal targets for D-optimality Φ_D and A-optimality Φ_A (see Table 1.1) are respectively:

$$\pi_B^* = 1/2$$

and

$$\pi_N^* = \frac{\sqrt{Var[Y_A]}}{\sqrt{Var[Y_A]} + \sqrt{Var[Y_B]}}.$$

From now on we always assume "the-larger-the-θ-the better" scenario, namely A is better than B if $\theta_A > \theta_B$. Given an optimality criterion Φ, we write $\Phi\left[\mathbf{M}^{-1}(\theta_A; \theta_B \mid \pi)\right] = \Phi(\pi)$ with a slight abuse of notation. Since we always deal with convex criteria, $\Phi(\pi)$ is also a convex function of π and in fact in all the cases of interest it will be strictly convex, so that there is a unique $\pi_{\mathcal{I}}^*$ satisfying (5.2).

Generally, $\lim_{\pi\to 0}\Phi(\pi) = \lim_{\pi\to 1}\Phi(\pi) = \infty$; in these cases the comparative experiment degenerates to observing just one treatment, which obviously makes treatment comparison impossible.

5.2.2 Ethically optimal targets

We now wish to deal with design optimality for purposes other than inference and, in particular, to introduce suitable "ethical criteria" aimed at measuring the ethical cost of the experiment. One of the most popular criteria in use in a clinical context is the loss due to the proportion of patients who receive the worse treatment, namely

$$\mathcal{E}(\pi) = \begin{cases} 1-\pi & \text{if } \theta_A > \theta_B, \\ \pi & \text{if } \theta_A < \theta_B. \end{cases} \tag{5.3}$$

This criterion is a linear function of the allocation proportion π to A (increasing or decreasing on the basis of the inferiority/superiority of treatment A), and is clearly minimized by assigning all the statistical units to the better treatment, so the optimal ethical target is simply

$$\pi^*_{\mathcal{E}} = \frac{1}{2} + \frac{\operatorname{sgn}(\theta_A - \theta_B)}{2}. \tag{5.4}$$

It goes without saying that target $\pi^*_{\mathcal{E}}$ is a priori unknown, it depends only on the sign of the difference of treatment effects (but not on the nuisance parameters, even if present). When $\theta_A = \theta_B$ there is no longer a worse treatment; so (5.3) no longer depends on the design and every target allocation could be considered as ethically optimal.

For binary responses another possible measure of ethical cost considered by several authors (see Rosenberger et al. (2001a)) is the total expected proportion of failures

$$\tilde{\mathcal{E}}(\pi) = \pi q_A + (1-\pi) q_B, \tag{5.5}$$

which for $p_A \neq p_B$ is simply a linear transformation of $\mathcal{E}(\pi)$. To see this, let $q_{\min} = \min\{q_A, q_B\}$ and $q_{\max} = \max\{q_A, q_B\}$, then $\tilde{\mathcal{E}}(\pi) \in [q_{\min}; q_{\max}]$ and

$$\frac{\tilde{\mathcal{E}}(\pi) - q_{\min}}{q_{\max} - q_{\min}} = \frac{\pi q_A + (1-\pi) q_B - q_{\min}}{|p_A - p_B|} = \mathcal{E}(\pi). \tag{5.6}$$

Therefore, criterion (5.5) provides the same information about $\mathcal{E}(\pi)$ on a different scale. The change of scale depends on the parameters.

In practice, we would most likely wish to simultaneously minimize both the ethical cost and the inferential loss. However, these are in general conflicting aims. For instance, from (1.27) and (1.30) it is evident that the ethically optimal target $\pi^*_{\mathcal{E}}$ induces the worst possible scenario from an inferential viewpoint, leading to an infinite loss of information. The problem is how to achieve a good trade-off between inferential goals and ethical demands; we shall deal with this in Section 5.4.

5.3 Non-admissible targets

With just one optimality criterion, a treatment allocation proportion will be preferred to another one if it improves the value of the chosen criterion. However, since target allocations are in general functions of the parameters $\gamma = (\gamma_A; \gamma_B)^t$, whether or not one allocation is to be preferred to another may depend on the unknown state of nature. With several criteria in multi-objective experiments, a given treatment allocation will be preferred to another if it represents an improvement with respect to at least one of the criteria, guaranteeing at the same time non-inferior performances with respect to all the others. This introduces a preference ordering among the targets which is clearly partial and in general two targets will not be comparable. And again, this preference may also depend on the unknown values of the parameters.

Within this framework, Baldi Antognini and Giovagnoli (2010) have introduced a mild condition, called *admissibility*, to describe target allocations that cannot be improved upon with respect to all the chosen design criteria for all the values of the unknown parameters.

Definition 5.1 *A target π is said to be* ***non-admissible*** *if for some values of the parameters γ there exist better allocations with respect to all the adopted criteria.*

Thus, after choosing the appropriate design criteria in a given experimental context, it is sensible to restrict our attention only to the admissible targets. More specifically, in the context of just two treatments if Φ is the chosen criterion for information loss, a given target is admissible if there does not exist another allocation which, for some values of the unknown parameters, is both more informative with respect to Φ and, at the same time, has more ethical appeal.

Definition 5.2 *(Baldi Antognini and Giovagnoli (2010)) An allocation π is said to be* ***admissible*** *with respect to the chosen pair of criteria $(\Phi, \mathcal{E})$ if there does not exist another allocation $\dot{\pi}$ such that*

$$\Phi(\pi) \geq \Phi(\dot{\pi}) \quad \text{and} \quad \mathcal{E}(\pi) \geq \mathcal{E}(\dot{\pi}), \tag{5.7}$$

for some values of γ_A and γ_B, where at least one inequality is strict.

Some remarks:

- the inferentially optimal target $\pi_{\mathcal{I}}^*$ in (5.2) and the optimal ethical target $\pi_{\mathcal{E}}^*$ in (5.4) are always admissible, since they cannot be improved with respect to the chosen information criterion Φ and ethical measure $\mathcal{E}$, respectively;
- if $\theta_A = \theta_B$ then every allocation becomes equivalent w.r.t $\mathcal{E}(\cdot)$, so the admissible target is unique and coincides with $\pi_{\mathcal{I}}^*$ in (5.2);
- in the context of binary trials, since criterion $\tilde{\mathcal{E}}$ in (5.5) is an increasing linear transformation of $\mathcal{E}$, a target is admissible with respect to $(\Phi, \mathcal{E})$ if and only if it is admissible with respect to $(\Phi, \tilde{\mathcal{E}})$.

A necessary and sufficient condition for admissibility of a target with respect to a pair $(\Phi, \mathcal{E})$ is

Proposition 5.1 *A target π is admissible with respect to $(\Phi, \mathcal{E})$ if and only if*

$$(\pi - \pi_{\mathcal{I}}^*)(\theta_A - \theta_B) \geq 0\,, \qquad \forall(\gamma_A, \gamma_B) \tag{5.8}$$

where $\pi_{\mathcal{I}}^*$ is the optimal inferential target minimizing Φ.

The proof of Proposition 5.1 was given by Baldi Antognini and Giovagnoli (2010) for binary responses and is identical in the more general case too. As a special case of Proposition 5.1 we get:

Corollary 5.1 *A target π is admissible with respect to the pair $(\Phi_D, \mathcal{E})$ (D-admissible for short) if and only if it assigns the majority of subjects to the better treatment, i.e.*

$$\left(\pi - \frac{1}{2}\right)(\theta_A - \theta_B) \geq 0\,, \qquad \forall(\gamma_A, \gamma_B); \tag{5.9}$$

whereas π is admissible with respect to the pair $(\Phi_A, \mathcal{E})$ (A-admissible for short) if and only if

$$(\pi - \pi_N^*)(\theta_A - \theta_B) \geq 0\,, \qquad \forall(\gamma_A, \gamma_B). \tag{5.10}$$

A straightforward consequence is also

Corollary 5.2 *For binary responses, all targets of the form*

$$\frac{p_A^z/q_A^t}{p_A^z/q_A^t + p_B^z/q_B^t} \tag{5.11}$$

where z and t are real numbers, are D-admissible if and only if $z \geq 0$ and $t \geq 0$, since they assign the majority of subjects to the better treatment. They are A-admissible if and only if $z \geq 1/2$ and $t \geq -1/2$, since it is easy to check that

$$\left(\frac{p_A^z/q_A^t}{p_A^z/q_A^t + p_B^z/q_B^t} - \frac{\sqrt{p_A q_A}}{\sqrt{p_A q_A} + \sqrt{p_B q_B}}\right)(p_A - p_B) \geq 0, \qquad \forall(p_A, p_B).$$

Expression (5.11) above includes the target $\pi_{PW}^* = q_B/(q_A + q_B)$ when $z = 0$ and $t = 1$, the "dual" target $p_A/(p_A + p_B)$ ($z = 1$ and $t = 0$), the odds-based target ($z = 1$ and $t = 1$), the odds-ratio-based target ($z = 2$ and $t = 2$) of Section 4.2.1 and, for $z = 1/2$ and $t = 0$, the target allocation proposed by Rosenberger et al. (2001a)

$$\pi_R^* = \frac{\sqrt{p_A}}{\sqrt{p_A} + \sqrt{p_B}}. \tag{5.12}$$

When $z = 1/2$ and $t = -1/2$, target (5.11) becomes Neyman's allocation.

Example 5.1 *For binary outcomes and Φ_D the D-optimality criterion, the following results hold:*

i) *the Neyman allocation π_N^* is non-admissible with respect to the pair $(\Phi_D, \mathcal{E})$, since from (5.9) $\pi_N^* < 1/2$ when $p_A > p_B$ and $p_A + p_B > 1$, namely it is sometimes dominated by the balanced target.*

ii) *the target π^*_{PW} is D-admissible;*

iii) *the target π^*_{dawd} discussed in Chapter 4 is D-admissible,*

Example 5.2 *For binary outcomes and Φ_A the A-optimality criterion, the following results hold:*

i) *the balanced allocation is non-admissible with respect to the pair $(\Phi_A, \mathcal{E})$;*

ii) *the Play-the-Winner target $\pi^*_{PW} = q_B/(q_A + q_B)$ is non-admissible;*

iii) *the target π^*_{dawd} is non-admissible, since it is dominated by the Neyman target π^*_N for some values of (p_A, p_B) (see Baldi Antognini and Giovagnoli (2010) for details);*

iv) *the target allocation π^*_R in (5.12) is A-admissible.*

Example 5.3 *For normally distributed responses with $\mu_A, \mu_B > 0$,*

i) *the target*

$$\pi = \frac{\mu_A}{\mu_A + \mu_B} \tag{5.13}$$

is D-admissible because it assigns the better treatment to the majority of subjects, and is non-admissible with respect to $(\Phi_A, \mathcal{E})$, since

$$\text{if} \quad \frac{\sigma_A}{\sigma_B} > \frac{\mu_A}{\mu_B} > 1 \quad \Rightarrow \quad \frac{\mu_A}{\mu_A + \mu_B} < \frac{\sigma_A}{\sigma_A + \sigma_B},$$

namely (5.13) is sometimes dominated by the Neyman allocation π^*_N;

ii) *the target*

$$\pi = \frac{\mu_A \sigma_A}{\mu_A \sigma_A + \mu_B \sigma_B} \tag{5.14}$$

is A-admissible since from (5.10)

$$\left(\frac{\mu_A \sigma_A}{\mu_A \sigma_A + \mu_B \sigma_B} - \frac{\sigma_A}{\sigma_A + \sigma_B} \right) (\mu_A - \mu_B) \geq 0 \,, \qquad \forall \mu_A, \mu_B, \sigma^2_A, \sigma^2_B > 0;$$

whereas it is non-admissible with respect to the pair $(\Phi_D, \mathcal{E})$, since it is dominated by the balanced allocation if

$$1 < \frac{\mu_A}{\mu_B} < \frac{\sigma_B}{\sigma_A}.$$

As shown by Examples 5.1 and 5.2, there are target allocations that are simultaneously admissible with respect to different inferential criteria. In Section 5.5 we will show how to derive target allocations that are admissible with respect to a chosen pair of criteria.

5.4 Multi-objective optimal targets: The constrained optimization approach

There are two available approaches in the literature for deriving multipurpose optimal target allocations of the treatments, namely constrained optimization and compound optimization. Here we deal with just two experimental goals suitably formalized into two different design criteria, which for the moment we shall keep very general, although we are motivated by the case in which one is a measure of inferential loss and the other one an indicator of ethical loss, as in Sections 5.2 and 5.3. An extension to the case of several criteria is discussed in Clyde and Chaloner (1996).

For combination purposes, all criteria need to be standardized first, to put them on a comparable scale. The standardized criteria $\Psi_1(\cdot)$ and $\Psi_2(\cdot)$ will be chosen to lie in [0;1], namely $\Psi_1, \Psi_2 : [0;1] \to [0;1]$ will be two non-negative functions of π to be minimized (as previously, for ease of notation we neglect the dependence on the unknown model parameters).

Adopting a constrained optimization approach, the problem consists in finding the allocation proportion that optimizes either criterion under a suitable constraint on the other. From a mathematical viewpoint it is not necessary that both Ψ_1 and Ψ_2 be measures ranging in the same interval $[0;1]$, but it is important always to refer to the standardized versions of the chosen design criteria since the adoption of non-standardized criteria could cause some problems, as we shall discuss in Remark 5.1 and at the end of the section. Formally, the constrained optimal target π_C^* is obtained by solving the following optimization problem:

$$\begin{cases} \text{minimize} & \Psi_2(\pi), \\ \text{subject to} & \Psi_1(\pi) \leq C, \end{cases} \tag{5.15}$$

where $C \in (0;1)$ is a given constant chosen in advance representing the maximum loss of efficiency for the primary criterion, say Ψ_1, that we are willing to accept (the degenerate case $C = 1$ is excluded, since it corresponds to assuming just a single design criterion). Thus, for any given choice of C the problem is i) finding the set S_C of allocations that guarantees a prescribed level of efficiency with respect to Ψ_1 and then ii) finding the target that minimizes Ψ_2 over S_C (instead of the entire design region $[0;1]$).

Clearly, the choice of the maximum loss C for criterion Ψ_1 is crucial and, even if not explicitly stated in the optimization problem (5.15), it clearly induces a corresponding *weight* of criterion Ψ_2; thus, C should be interpreted as the relative importance of Ψ_1 with respect to Ψ_2.

Usually the two criteria are not exchangeable: the experimental goal expressed by Ψ_1 is often considered more important than that of Ψ_2 (as, for instance, in the classical hypothesis testing approach of Neyman and Pearson). Only in the case of linearity of at least one of the two criteria, is problem (5.15) equivalent to minimizing $\Psi_1(\cdot)$ under a constraint on $\Psi_2(\cdot)$.

If both Ψ_1 and Ψ_2 are convex and differentiable functions of π, (5.15) is a convex optimization problem and therefore the optimal solution π_C^* is unique. Indeed, since Ψ_1 is continuous and strictly convex, for any given $C \in (0;1)$ the set S_C is a compact subinterval of $[0;1]$, so that π_C^* can usually be found by standard differentiation techniques.

Suppose now that the chosen criteria are measures of inferential loss Φ and ethical loss $\mathcal{E}$, respectively, as in Section 5.2. Let $\pi_{\mathcal{I}}^*$ in (5.2) be the inferentially optimal target minimizing Φ, then the standardized loss of inferential efficiency can be measured by

$$\Psi_1(\pi) = 1 - \frac{\Phi(\pi_{\mathcal{I}}^*)}{\Phi(\pi)}; \tag{5.16}$$

whereas we can set $\Psi_2(\pi) = \mathcal{E}(\pi)$ directly, due to the fact that the ethical loss lies in $[0;1]$. Since $\mathcal{E}(\cdot)$ is linear in π, there exists a unique constrained optimal target π_C^* satisfying

$$\begin{cases} \text{minimize} & \mathcal{E}(\pi), \\ \text{subject to} & 1 - \frac{\Phi(\pi_{\mathcal{I}}^*)}{\Phi(\pi)} \leq C. \end{cases} \tag{5.17}$$

Furthermore, this target π_C^* is always admissible with respect to the pair $(\Phi; \mathcal{E})$. Indeed, since Φ is continuous and strictly convex, for any given $C \in (0;1)$ we have that $\pi_{\mathcal{I}}^* \in S_C \subset [0;1]$ and therefore admissibility follows directly from Corollary 5.1, because $\mathcal{E}(\pi)$ is strictly decreasing if $\theta_A > \theta_B$ and strictly increasing when $\theta_A < \theta_B$.

Remark 5.1 *Letting $\tilde{C} = \Phi(\pi_{\mathcal{I}}^*)/(1-C)$, the optimization problem (5.17) can be rewritten as follows*

$$\begin{cases} \textit{minimize} & \mathcal{E}(\pi), \\ \textit{subject to} & \Phi(\pi) \leq \tilde{C}. \end{cases}$$

Thus, it is also possible to take into account design criteria that are not standardized, but if so the threshold should generally depend on the unknown parameters.

Example 5.4 *Consider a trial with normal responses $N(\mu_j; \sigma_j^2)$ $(j = A, B)$ and assume that Φ_D in (1.28) and $\mathcal{E}$ in (5.3) are the criteria of interest for information and ethics, respectively. Recalling that the target minimizing the D-optimality criterion is the balanced one $\pi_{\mathcal{I}}^* = 1/2$, the loss of inferential efficiency can be measured by*

$$\Psi_1(\pi) = 1 - \frac{\Phi_D(\pi_{\mathcal{I}}^*)}{\Phi_D(\pi)} = 1 - \frac{4\sigma_A^2\sigma_B^2}{\left[\frac{\sigma_A^2\sigma_B^2}{\pi(1-\pi)}\right]} = 1 - 4\pi(1-\pi),$$

so that the optimization problem consists in finding the allocation proportion π_C^* solving

$$\begin{cases} \textit{minimize} & \mathcal{E}(\pi), \\ \textit{subject to} & (1-2\pi)^2 \leq C, \end{cases}$$

for a prescribed maximum tolerated loss of inferential efficiency $C \in (0;1)$. *Due to the constraint,* $S_C = \left[\frac{1-\sqrt{C}}{2}; \frac{1+\sqrt{C}}{2}\right]$ *and the solution is*

$$\pi_C^* = \frac{1+\sqrt{C}\cdot sgn(\mu_A - \mu_B)}{2}, \tag{5.18}$$

since the ethical loss $\mathcal{E}$ *is decreasing (respectively increasing) in* π *if* $\mu_A > \mu_B$ $(\mu_A < \mu_B)$*. It is easy to show that* π_C^* *in (5.18) always assigns the majority of subjects to the better treatment, namely it is admissible with respect to* $(\Phi_D; \mathcal{E})$.

Note that in Example 5.4 the optimal constrained target π_C^* depends on the unknown parameters μ_A and μ_B only through the sign of $\mu_A - \mu_B$ and not on its magnitude; thus, the amount of the ethical skew depends only on C. Assuming $\mu_A > \mu_B$, Figure 5.1 shows the behaviour of the optimal constrained target π_C^* in (5.18) as C varies. For instance, if we set $C = 0.01$ (i.e. the inferential demand is extremely important with respect to ethics) then $\pi_C^* = 0.55$, while $\pi_C^* = 0.75$ when $C = 0.25$.

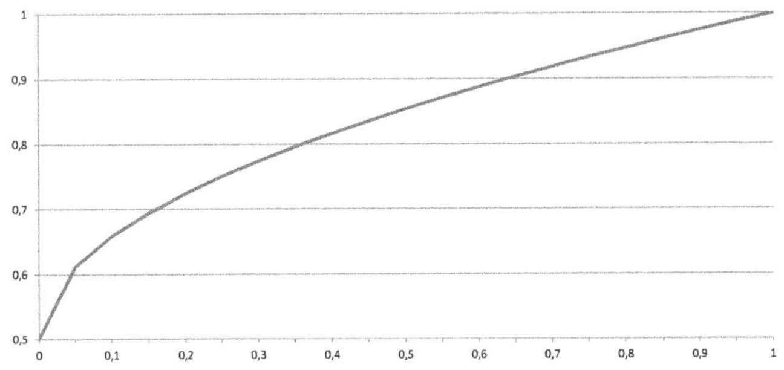

FIGURE 5.1: Optimal constrained target π_C^* in (5.18) as C varies in $(0;1)$.

As can be seen immediately, the major drawback of this approach is related to the definition of a suitable threshold C: ideally, C could be set to depend on the unknown parameters; for instance, in Example 5.4 if we let $C \geq (\sigma_A - \sigma_B)^2/(\sigma_A + \sigma_B)^2$ then the corresponding optimal constrained target π_C^* is also admissible with respect to the pair $(\Phi_A; \mathcal{E})$. However, this choice has neither a clear interpretation nor a mathematical justification.

Example 5.5 *Consider a binary response trial and let* $\mathcal{E}$ *in (5.3) and* Φ_A *in (1.30)* *be the chosen criteria. Since the inferentially optimal target is the Neyman allocation* π_N^*, *then* $\Phi_A(\pi_N^*) = \left(\sqrt{p_Aq_A} + \sqrt{p_Bq_B}\right)^2$ *and therefore the optimization problem is*

$$\begin{cases} \textit{minimize} & \mathcal{E}(\pi) \\ \textit{subject to} & 1 - \frac{\left(\sqrt{p_Aq_A}+\sqrt{p_Bq_B}\right)^2}{\frac{p_Aq_A}{\pi}+\frac{p_Bq_B}{1-\pi}} \leq C. \end{cases}$$

Thus, S_C *is given by*

$$\left[\frac{\sqrt{p_Aq_A}}{\sqrt{p_Aq_A}+\sqrt{p_Bq_B}}(1-C)+\frac{C}{2} \pm \frac{\sqrt{C^2\left(\sqrt{p_Aq_A}-\sqrt{p_Bq_B}\right)^2+4C\sqrt{p_Aq_Ap_Bq_B}}}{2(\sqrt{p_Aq_A}+\sqrt{p_Bq_B})}\right]$$

and the optimal constrained target is

$$\pi_C^* = \frac{\sqrt{p_Aq_A}}{\sqrt{p_Aq_A}+\sqrt{p_Bq_B}}(1-C)+\frac{C}{2}+$$
$$+\left[\frac{\sqrt{C^2\left(\sqrt{p_Aq_A}-\sqrt{p_Bq_B}\right)^2+4C\sqrt{p_Aq_Ap_Bq_B}}}{2(\sqrt{p_Aq_A}+\sqrt{p_Bq_B})}\right] sgn(p_A-p_B),$$

which is admissible with respect to $(\Phi_A; \mathcal{E})$; *indeed, from Corollary 5.1, it can be shown after tedious algebra that*

$$\left(\pi_C^* - \frac{\sqrt{p_Aq_A}}{\sqrt{p_Aq_A}+\sqrt{p_Bq_B}}\right)(p_A-p_B) \geq 0, \quad \textit{for all } (p_A, p_B).$$

In the constrained approach, the choice of C is easy to interpret only when the design criteria express measures of efficiency, whereas adopting non-standardized indicators any choice of the threshold tends to be quite arbitrary and partially improper. Several authors have suggested target allocation of the treatments derived through non-standardized design criteria; see Rosenberger et al. (2001a), Biswas and Mandal (2007), Tymofyeyev et al. (2007), Jeon and Hu (2010), Biswas et al. (2011) and Sverdlov and Rosenberger (2013a). For binary response trials, Rosenberger et al. (2001a) consider the following optimization problem

$$\begin{cases} \text{minimize} & n[\pi q_A + (1-\pi)q_B], \\ \text{subject to} & n^{-1}\left(\frac{p_Aq_A}{\pi}+\frac{p_Bq_B}{1-\pi}\right) = \tilde{C}, \end{cases} \tag{5.19}$$

namely finding the target allocation that minimizes the total expected number of failures, subject to a suitable constraint on the variance of the estimated treatment difference. But the variance of the estimated treatment difference depends on the total sample size and the unknown parameters, so every choice of $\tilde{C}$ should itself be a function of n and (p_A, p_B).

From the constraint it follows that

$$n = \tilde{C}^{-1}\left(\frac{p_Aq_A}{\pi}+\frac{p_Bq_B}{1-\pi}\right), \tag{5.20}$$

so the authors obtain the target allocation π_R^* in (5.12). Unlike Examples 5.4 and 5.5, the constrained optimal target π_R^* does not depend on the prescribed threshold $\tilde{C}$. This is due to the fact that the effect of the constraint is incorporated into the sample size, namely this is an optimization problem in two variables and its solution is not just π_R^*, but the pair $(\pi_R^*; n^*)$, where from (5.20)

$$n^* = \tilde{C}^{-1}(\sqrt{p_A} + \sqrt{p_B})(q_A\sqrt{p_A} + q_B\sqrt{p_B}). \tag{5.21}$$

First of all observe that, since the constraint is related to the variance of the estimated treatment difference, at each step $n \geq 2$ (with at least one allocation to either treatment) we have

$$\frac{p_A q_A}{N_{An}} + \frac{p_B q_B}{N_{Bn}} \leq \frac{1}{4N_{An}} + \frac{1}{4N_{Bn}} \leq \frac{1}{2}$$

and thus any choice of $\tilde{C} > 1/2$ leads to a formal contradiction. Therefore $\tilde{C}$ should be set $\leq 1/2$; however, how much smaller than $\leq 1/2$ should it be? From (5.21), the optimal sample size satisfies $n^* \leq \tilde{C}^{-1}$ (the maximum value $n^* = \tilde{C}^{-1}$ can be obtained only if $p_A = p_B = 1/2$). For instance, if we set $\tilde{C} = 0.1$, then $n^* \simeq 4$ for $p_A = p_B = 0.9$ and $n^* \simeq 7$ for $(p_A, p_B) = (0.9; 0.6)$; while letting $\tilde{C} = 0.05$, then $n^* \simeq 7$ or $\simeq 14$ if $p_A = p_B = 0.9$ or $(p_A, p_B) = (0.9; 0.6)$, respectively. It is evident that these sample sizes are a long way away from guaranteeing the convergence of a response-adaptive design implemented for targeting π_R^*. A possible way to overcome these drawbacks is to let $\tilde{C}$ be a function of the unknown parameters and the sample size, leading to a design criterion based on efficiency.

5.5 Multi-objective optimal targets: The combined optimization approach

A combined optimization approach means specifying an appropriate compound criterion that acts as a trade-off between the different criteria of interest, after standardization. The standardized criteria $\Psi_1(\pi)$ and $\Psi_2(\pi)$ lie in [0;1]. A natural compromise consists in taking a convex combination of them, for instance a weighted arithmetic mean or weighted harmonic mean, with suitable weights.

Starting with the simplest scenario, we look at the following combination

$$\Psi_\omega(\pi) = (1-\omega)\,\Psi_1(\pi) + \omega\Psi_2(\pi), \tag{5.22}$$

as the compromise criterion to be minimized, where the weights ω and $1-\omega$ in $(0;1)$ represent the relative importance of Ψ_1 (e.g. the inferential loss) and Ψ_2 (e.g. the ethical loss). We rule out the degenerate cases $\omega = 0$ or 1 corresponding to assuming just one criterion. Instead of ω and $1-\omega$ it is sometimes easier to use the odds $\omega/(1-\omega)$. Thus the optimal combined target is given by

$$\pi_\omega^* = \arg\min_\pi \Psi_\omega(\pi)$$

and if both Ψ_1 and Ψ_2 are strictly convex, then $\Psi_\omega(\pi)$ is also strictly convex and therefore the solution π^*_ω is unique. If in addition Ψ_1 and Ψ_2 are differentiable functions, the optimal combined target can be found by differentiation of Φ_ω with respect to π, i.e., looking for a solution in $(0;1)$ of the equation

$$\left(\frac{\omega}{1-\omega}\right)\frac{\partial\Psi_2(\pi)}{\partial\pi}+\frac{\partial\Psi_1(\pi)}{\partial\pi}=0. \tag{5.23}$$

For instance, if we let $\mathcal{E}$ in (5.3) and Ψ_1 in (5.16) be the standardized criteria of interest, the compound criterion is

$$\Psi_\omega(\pi)=\omega\mathcal{E}(\pi)+(1-\omega)\left(1-\frac{\Phi(\pi^*_\mathcal{I})}{\Phi(\pi)}\right). \tag{5.24}$$

If the function $1/\Phi(\pi)$ is strictly concave, then $\Psi_\omega(\pi)$ is strictly convex, so there is a unique combined optimal target
indexkeywordsoptimal combined target $\pi^*_\omega\in(0;1)$ solving the equation

$$\left(\frac{\omega}{1-\omega}\right)\frac{\operatorname{sgn}(\theta_A-\theta_B)}{\Phi(\pi^*_\mathcal{I})}+\frac{\partial\left[1/\Phi(\pi)\right]}{\partial\pi}=0. \tag{5.25}$$

Whatever the choice of the weight ω, the optimal combined target π^*_ω solving (5.25) is always admissible with respect to $(\Phi;\mathcal{E})$. Indeed, letting

$$h(\pi)=\frac{\partial\left[1/\Phi(\pi)\right]}{\partial\pi}=-\frac{\left[\frac{\partial\Phi(\pi)}{\partial\pi}\right]}{[\Phi(\pi)]^2},$$

the concavity of $1/\Phi(\pi)$ implies that $h(\cdot)$ is strictly decreasing and furthermore $h(\pi^*_\mathcal{I})=0$. Thus, from (5.23) it is quite evident that $\pi^*_\omega>\pi^*_\mathcal{I}$ if $\theta_A>\theta_B$ and $\pi^*_\omega<\pi^*_\mathcal{I}$ if $\theta_A<\theta_B$.

5.5.1 The choice of the weights

As regards the choice of ω and $1-\omega$, they can be set as fixed constants. Otherwise, we may want to choose them according to the true values of the unknown model parameters, due to the fact that more attention must be paid to inference when θ_A and θ_B are close, since it is harder to discriminate between the two treatments. Care for the other goal could be more crucial, especially from an ethical point of view, if the treatment effects differ in a substantial way.

If so, we shall assume ω to be a continuous function of the unknown parameters γ_A and γ_B, i.e.,

$$\omega=\omega(\gamma_A;\gamma_B):\Omega\to(0;1),$$

satisfying the following conditions:

- D1 the function ω should deal with the treatments symmetrically;
- D2 ω should be non-decreasing in the absolute difference $|\theta_A-\theta_B|$ between the treatment effects.

Generally, a suitable choice of the weight function will depend on the given applied context. For instance, in Phase III trials the experimenters often have some information about the treatment effects gathered from previous stages, so more attention could be devoted to inference (provided that the ethical costs are not prohibitive, such as severe adverse effects on patients) and ω can be chosen to be slowly increasing. Moreover, since in clinical situations small differences between the treatment effects are often assumed to be negligible up to a given threshold ς (the minimal clinically important difference), and then to increase rapidly, we may assume $\omega(x) = 0$ for $x \leq \varsigma$ and $\omega(x) \rightarrow 1$ very quickly as x grows.

Example 5.6 *In a normal response trial with $N(\mu_j; \sigma_j^2)$ $(j = A, B)$ with Φ_D in (1.28) and $\mathcal{E}$ in (5.3) the criteria of interest for information and ethics, respectively, equation (5.25) becomes*

$$\left(\frac{\omega}{1-\omega}\right)\frac{sgn(\mu_A - \mu_B)}{4\sigma_A^2\sigma_B^2} + \frac{1-2\pi}{\sigma_A^2\sigma_B^2} = 0,$$

so that the corresponding optimal combined target is

$$\pi_\omega^* = \frac{1}{2} + sgn(\mu_A - \mu_B)\min\left\{\frac{1}{8}\left(\frac{\omega}{1-\omega}\right), \frac{1}{2}\right\}. \tag{5.26}$$

Note that π_ω^* in (5.26) is independent of σ_A^2 and σ_B^2 and if $\omega < 4/5$ then

$$\pi_\omega^* = \frac{1}{2} + \text{sgn}(\mu_A - \mu_B)\frac{1}{8}\left(\frac{\omega}{1-\omega}\right) \in (0,1). \tag{5.27}$$

If $\omega \geq 4/5$, π_ω^* will assign all the subjects to the better treatment. Thus, in order to obtain a non-degenerate optimal combined target, the ethical weight should be less than 80%.

This raises the question of how we can choose ω in an optimal way for Example 5.6. To answer this question, we can compare π_ω^* and the balanced design $\pi_\mathcal{I}^* = 1/2$ (that can be obtained by letting $\omega \rightarrow 0$) by taking into account the loss of inferential efficiency associated with the D-optimality criterion, namely

$$\Psi_1(\pi) = 1 - \frac{\Phi(\pi_\mathcal{I}^*)}{\Phi(\pi)} = (1-2\pi_\omega^*)^2 = \begin{cases} \left[\frac{\omega}{4(1-\omega)}\right]^2 & \omega < 4/5, \\ 1 & \omega \geq 4/5, \end{cases} \tag{5.28}$$

and the "ethical efficiency" measured by the relative percentage of subjects assigned to the better treatment by π_ω^* than by the balanced design, namely

$$\text{sgn}(\mu_A - \mu_B)(2\pi_\omega^* - 1) = \begin{cases} \frac{\omega}{4(1-\omega)} & \omega < 4/5, \\ 1 & \omega \geq 4/5. \end{cases} \tag{5.29}$$

The ethical gain and the inferential loss for the optimal combined target defined in (5.27) are compared in Table 5.1.

TABLE 5.1: Percentage of relative ethical gain and of relative loss of inferential efficiency for π_ω^* in (5.27) with respect to the balanced target as ω varies when $\mu_A > \mu_B$.

ω	π_ω^*	% ethical gain in (5.29)	% inferential loss in (5.28)
$\to 0$	$\to 0.5$	$\to 0$	$\to 0$
0.1	0.51	2.8	0.1
0.2	0.53	6.3	0.4
0.3	0.55	10.7	1.2
0.4	0.58	16.7	2.8
0.5	0.63	25.0	6.3
0.6	0.69	37.5	14.1
2/3	0.75	50.0	25.0
0.7	0.79	58.3	34.0
0.8	1	100.0	100.0

From (5.28) and (5.29), both the ethical gain and the inferential loss degenerate to 1 when the ethical weight is greater than 80%, while for $\omega < 4/5$ the ethical gain induced by the optimal combined target is always greater than the inferential loss, with maximum difference at $\omega = 2/3$. Therefore, this value of the weight could be considered a suitable choice.

Another possibility is to let ω depend on the unknown model parameters. For instance, for normal responses we could choose

$$\omega = \frac{4}{5}\left(1 - e^{-\frac{|\mu_A-\mu_B|}{\sqrt{\sigma_A^2+\sigma_B^2}}}\right), \tag{5.30}$$

so that $\pi_\omega^* \neq 0, 1$. Letting $\mu_A > \mu_B$ (wlog), Table 5.2 shows the behaviour of the optimal combined target π_ω^* in (5.27) for possible values of $(\mu_A - \mu_B)/\sqrt{\sigma_A^2 + \sigma_B^2}$.

TABLE 5.2: Values of the optimum combined target π_ω^* in (5.27) with weight function ω in (5.30).

$\frac{\mu_A-\mu_B}{\sqrt{\sigma_A^2+\sigma_B^2}}$	ω	π_ω^*
$\to 0$	$\to 0$	0.500
0.25	0.18	0.527
0.50	0.31	0.557
0.75	0.42	0.591
1.00	0.51	0.628
1.50	0.62	0.705
3.00	0.76	0.896
$\to \infty$	$\to 0.8$	1.000

5.5.2 Combined optimization approach involving efficiencies

An alternative compromise criterion based on the efficiencies (instead of the loss of efficiencies) was suggested by Dette (1997)

$$\tilde{\Psi}_\omega(\pi) = \omega\left[\frac{1}{1-\Psi_2(\pi)}\right] + (1-\omega)\left[\frac{1}{1-\Psi_1(\pi)}\right], \tag{5.31}$$

which can be seen as the reciprocal of the weighted harmonic mean of the efficiencies $1-\Psi_1$ and $1-\Psi_2$ (see also Baldi Antognini and Giovagnoli (2010)). Clearly $\tilde{\Psi}_\omega$ should be minimized and when $\tilde{\Psi}_\omega(\pi)$ is a strictly convex differentiable function, the unique solution π^*_ω can be found by standard differentiation techniques. For instance, letting $\mathcal{E}$ and Φ be the usual criteria of ethical and inferential loss, the compound criterion in (5.31) becomes

$$\tilde{\Psi}_\omega(\pi) = \omega\left[\frac{1}{1-\mathcal{E}(\pi)}\right] + (1-\omega)\left[\frac{\Phi(\pi)}{\Phi(\pi^*_I)}\right],$$

which is strictly convex since $\mathcal{E}(\cdot)$ is linear. Thus, the unique optimal combined target π^*_ω is the solution in $(0;1)$ of the following equation

$$[1-\mathcal{E}(\pi)]^2\left(\frac{\partial\Phi(\pi)}{\partial\pi}\right) = \left(\frac{\omega}{1-\omega}\right)\Phi(\pi^*_I)\mathrm{sgn}(\theta_A-\theta_B) \tag{5.32}$$

and is admissible with respect to $(\Phi;\mathcal{E})$.

Example 5.7 *For a binary response trial suppose that Φ_D in (1.28) and $\mathcal{E}$ in (5.3) are the criteria of interest. Equation (5.32) becomes*

$$[1-\mathcal{E}(\pi)]^2\left(\frac{p_Aq_Ap_Bq_B(2\pi-1)}{\pi^2(1-\pi)^2}\right) = (4p_Aq_Ap_Bq_B)\left(\frac{\omega}{1-\omega}\right)sgn(p_A-p_B)$$

namely

$$[1-\mathcal{E}(\pi)]^2\left(\frac{2\pi-1}{\pi^2(1-\pi)^2}\right) = 4\left(\frac{\omega}{1-\omega}\right)sgn(p_A-p_B),$$

so that the corresponding optimal combined target is

$$\pi^*_\omega = \frac{1}{2} + \left[\frac{(\omega+1)-\sqrt{(3\omega+1)(1-\omega)}}{4\omega}\right]sgn(p_A-p_B). \tag{5.33}$$

This target always assigns more than half the subjects to the better treatment. If the ethical weight ω is independent of p_A and p_B, π^*_ω depends just on the sign of the difference p_A-p_B and not on the actual values of the treatment effects. Letting (wlog) $p_A>p_B$, Figure 5.2 shows the behaviour of the optimal combined target π^*_ω in (5.33) as ω varies in $(0;1)$.

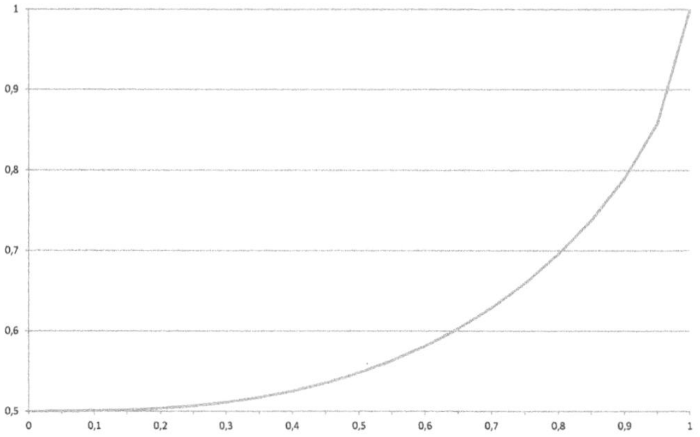

FIGURE 5.2: Optimal combined target π_ω^* in (5.33) as ω varies in $(0;1)$.

In the case of binary outcomes, if we chose $\tilde{\mathcal{E}}$ in (5.5) instead of $\mathcal{E}$, the ethical efficiency can be measured by

$$\frac{\tilde{\mathcal{E}}(\pi_{\mathcal{E}}^*)}{\tilde{\mathcal{E}}(\pi)} = \frac{q_{min}}{\tilde{\mathcal{E}}(\pi)},$$

so that the compound criterion becomes

$$\tilde{\Psi}_\omega(\pi) = \omega\left[\frac{\tilde{\mathcal{E}}(\pi)}{q_{min}}\right] + (1-\omega)\left[\frac{\Phi(\pi)}{\Phi(\pi_{\mathcal{I}}^*)}\right]. \tag{5.34}$$

This criterion is strictly convex and admits a unique minimum π_ω^* that solves

$$\frac{\partial\Phi(\pi)}{\partial\pi} = \left(\frac{\omega}{1-\omega}\right)\Phi(\pi_{\mathcal{I}}^*)\left(\frac{p_A - p_B}{q_{min}}\right), \tag{5.35}$$

and this optimal combined target is admissible with respect to $(\Phi;\tilde{\mathcal{E}})$.

Within this setting Baldi Antognini and Giovagnoli (2010) have proved a more general result about the connection between admissibility and compound optimal designs, showing that a target is admissible with respect to $(\Phi;\mathcal{E})$ (or, analogously, $(\Phi;\tilde{\mathcal{E}})$) if and only if it minimizes the compound criterion $\tilde{\Psi}_\omega(\pi)$ in (5.34) for a suitable choice of the weight function ω.

Example 5.8 *In a binary response trial, let Φ_A in (1.30) be the chosen inferential criterion. The optimal combined target is obtained by solving*

$$\frac{p_B q_B}{(1-\pi)^2} - \frac{p_A q_A}{\pi^2} = \left(\frac{\omega}{1-\omega}\right)(\sqrt{p_A q_A} + \sqrt{p_B q_B})^2\left(\frac{p_A - p_B}{q_{min}}\right). \tag{5.36}$$

Since the LHS of (5.36) is monotonic and, as $\pi \to 0$ and 1, the limits are $-\infty$ and $+\infty$, respectively, there is a unique solution in $(0,1)$. Unlike (5.33), in this case the optimal solution depends on the actual values of p_A and p_B and not just on the sign of their difference.

For any choice of ω, this combined target is clearly admissible with respect to $(\Phi_A; \mathcal{E})$; moreover, Baldi Antognini and Giovagnoli (2010) have shown that it is also admissible with respect to $(\Phi_D; \mathcal{E})$, namely the majority of subjects will receive the better treatment if the weight function is chosen so that $\omega(x,y) \geq 1/2$ when $x+y>1$.

Table 5.3 shows the values of the optimal combined targets that solve (5.36), corresponding to fixed weight $\omega = 1/2$ (denoted by $\pi^*_{\omega=1/2}$) and to $\omega = (\mid p_A - p_B \mid +1)/2$ (denoted by $\pi^*_{\omega_p}$) as p_A and p_B vary, also compared with Neyman's allocation π^*_N and the PW target π^*_{PW}.

TABLE 5.3: Values of Neyman's allocation π^*_N, PW target π^*_{PW} and the optimum combined target π^*_ω solving (5.36) with fixed weight $\omega = 0.5$ and $\omega = (\mid p_A - p_B \mid +1)/2$ as p_A and p_B vary.

p_A	p_B	$\pi^*_{\omega=1/2}$	$\pi^*_{\omega_p}$	π^*_N	π^*_{PW}
0.10	0.05	0.586	0.587	0.579	0.514
0.20	0.05	0.668	0.675	0.647	0.543
0.20	0.10	0.587	0.590	0.571	0.529
0.40	0.05	0.744	0.782	0.692	0.613
0.40	0.20	0.590	0.609	0.551	0.571
0.40	0.35	0.517	0.518	0.507	0.520
0.65	0.40	0.578	0.624	0.493	0.632
0.65	0.60	0.511	0.513	0.493	0.533
0.95	0.65	0.724	0.796	0.314	0.875
0.95	0.85	0.599	0.629	0.379	0.750

The targets $\pi^*_{\omega=1/2}$ and $\pi^*_{\omega_p}$ assign more patients to the better treatment, whereas the bottom part of Table 5.3 (outlined) shows the values of (p_A, p_B) for which the Neyman target penalizes the better treatment. Clearly the values of $\pi^*_{\omega=1/2}$ and $\pi^*_{\omega_p}$ are very close when $p_A \simeq p_B$.

5.5.3 Similarities and differences between constrained and combined optimization approaches

As shown by several authors (see Cook and Wong (1994), Clyde and Chaloner (1996), Baldi Antognini and Zagoraiou (2012)), constrained optimal designs and compound optimal designs are closely related. In point of fact, under the standard hypothesis of convexity and differentiability of the chosen efficiency measures, these two approaches are equivalent, namely every constrained optimal target allocation π^*_C can be viewed as the solution of a combined optimization problem with a suitable choice of the weights and vice versa.

For instance, the constrained optimization problem (5.19) can be simply rewritten as

$$\begin{cases} \text{minimize} & n\tilde{\mathcal{E}}(\pi), \\ \text{subject to} & \Phi_A(\pi) = n\tilde{C}, \end{cases} \quad \text{i.e.} \quad \begin{cases} \text{minimize} & \Phi_A(\pi)\tilde{\mathcal{E}}(\pi)\tilde{C}^{-1}, \\ \text{subject to} & n = \Phi_A(\pi)\tilde{C}^{-1}, \end{cases}$$

that is equivalent to finding the target allocation minimizing the product $\Phi_A(\pi)\tilde{\mathcal{E}}(\pi)$, since $\tilde{C}$ does not depend on π. Thus, the target allocation π_R^* in (5.12) could also be viewed as the solution of a compound optimization problem with a compound criterion given by the geometric mean of the chosen criteria (with equal weights).

Generally, the optimal target allocations derived by these approaches will depend on:

- the chosen criteria (as well as the selected compromise function in the compound framework);
- the relative importance of the two different goals, which must be chosen by the experimenter;
- the unknown model parameters.

If compared with compound optimization, the constrained approach is quite difficult to solve analytically, especially when both criteria are complicated non-linear functions. Furthermore, its applicability is strictly related to the identification of a suitable threshold C.

On the other hand, adopting the compound approach in general the optimization problem is easy to solve. Moreover, the possibility of modeling the weight ω as a function of the unknown model parameters introduces greater flexibility and also allows one to obtain optimal combined target that are simultaneously admissible with respect to both $(\Phi_A; \mathcal{E})$ and $(\Phi_D; \mathcal{E})$.

5.6 The case of several treatments

5.6.1 Inferential and ethical targets for v treatments

Taking now into account the case of $v \geq 2$ treatments, let $\boldsymbol{\theta} = (\theta_1, \ldots, \theta_v)^t$ be the vector of unknown treatment effects and $\boldsymbol{\pi}_n = (\pi_{n1}, \ldots, \pi_{nv})^t$ represent the allocation proportions to the treatments after n assignments, where clearly $\sum_{j=1}^{v} \pi_{nj} = 1$.

Let the inferentially optimal target be $\boldsymbol{\pi}_I^*$, namely the allocation vector minimizing $\Phi\left[\mathbf{M}^{-1}(\boldsymbol{\theta} \mid \boldsymbol{\pi})\right]$ for a suitably chosen convex criterion Φ. Of special interest is the case of the comparison of $v-1$ treatments with the remaining one (a control), so if we set $\mathbf{I}_v$ to be the v-dim identity matrix and $\mathbf{1}_v$ the v-dim vector of ones, then an appropriate matrix of contrasts is for instance $\mathbf{L} = [\mathbf{1}_{v-1} : \mathbf{I}_{v-1}]^t$, the matrix of elementary contrasts with respect to treatment T_1. The contrasts can be written as $\mathbf{L}^t\boldsymbol{\theta} = (\theta_1 - \theta_2; \ldots; \theta_1 - \theta_v)^t$, so beside D- and A-optimality, other criteria of interest are L-optimality and D_L-optimality (see Appendix A):

$$\Phi_{D_L}(\boldsymbol{\pi}) = \det[\mathbf{L}^t\mathbf{M}^{-1}(\boldsymbol{\theta} \mid \boldsymbol{\pi})\mathbf{L}] \text{ and } \Phi_L(\boldsymbol{\pi}) = \mathrm{tr}[\mathbf{L}^t\mathbf{M}^{-1}(\boldsymbol{\theta} \mid \boldsymbol{\pi})\mathbf{L}], \tag{5.37}$$

namely D- and A-optimality applied to the transformed information matrix (Atkinson, 1982; Wong and Zhu, 2008):

$$\mathbf{L}^t\mathbf{M}^{-1}(\boldsymbol{\theta} \mid \boldsymbol{\pi})\mathbf{L} = \frac{Var[Y_{T_1}]}{\pi_1}\mathbf{1}_{v-1}\mathbf{1}_{v-1}^t + \mathrm{diag}\left(\frac{Var[Y_{T_2}]}{\pi_2}; \ldots; \frac{Var[Y_{T_v}]}{\pi_v}\right). \tag{5.38}$$

As regards the "ethical criteria", measure (5.3) can be naturally extended to the case of v treatment by the proportion of patients who do not receive the best treatment(s)

$$\mathcal{E}(\boldsymbol{\pi}) = \sum_{j=1}^{v} \pi_j \mathrm{sgn}\left(\theta_{\max} - \theta_j\right), \tag{5.39}$$

where $\theta_{\max} = \max\{\theta_1, \ldots, \theta_v\}$. Note that criterion (5.39) considers only the superiority or inferiority of every treatment and does not take into account the different ethical gains induced by the magnitude $\theta_{\max} - \theta_j$ of the relative efficacy of each treatment. A modified version of criterion (5.39) that is able to discriminate between different ethical gains will be discussed in Section 6.5.

For binary responses, if we let $\boldsymbol{q} = (q_1, \ldots, q_v)^t$, the expected proportion of failures is

$$\tilde{\mathcal{E}}(\boldsymbol{\pi}) = \boldsymbol{\pi}^t\boldsymbol{q} \in [q_{\min}; q_{\max}]. \tag{5.40}$$

However, contrary to (5.6), if we standardize $\tilde{\mathcal{E}}(\boldsymbol{\pi})$ by letting

$$\frac{\tilde{\mathcal{E}}(\boldsymbol{\pi}) - q_{\min}}{q_{\max} - q_{\min}} = \sum_{j=1}^{v} \pi_j \left(\frac{p_{\max} - p_j}{p_{\max} - p_{\min}}\right) \qquad (\text{with } q_{\max} \neq q_{\min}),$$

it does not correspond to (5.39) since

$$\mathcal{E}(\boldsymbol{\pi}) = \sum_{j=1}^{v} \pi_j \mathrm{sgn}\left(p_{\max} - p_j\right) = \sum_{j=1}^{v} \pi_j \,\mathrm{sgn}\left(\frac{p_{\max} - p_j}{p_{\max} - p_{\min}}\right),$$

namely $\tilde{\mathcal{E}}$ accounts for the different treatment effects by re-scaling each p_j in terms of its relative inefficacy, whereas $\mathcal{E}$ can only distinguish whether a given treatment is the best one or not.

Clearly, both criteria (5.39) and (5.40) are linear functions minimized by the target $\boldsymbol{\pi}_{\mathcal{E}}^*$ that assigns all the subjects to the best treatment; when such treatment is not unique, $\boldsymbol{\pi}_{\mathcal{E}}^*$ could be replaced by any convex combination of allocations to all the best treatments.

In the case of several treatments, the following extension of Proposition 5.1 makes it easy to check the admissibility of a given target:

Proposition 5.2 *Let Φ be a strictly convex information criterion. A target $\boldsymbol{\pi}$ is admissible with respect to the pair $(\Phi_{\mathcal{I}}; \tilde{\mathcal{E}})$ if and only if*

$$\boldsymbol{\theta}^t\left(\boldsymbol{\pi}-\boldsymbol{\pi}_{\mathcal{I}}^*\right) \geq 0\,, \qquad \forall \boldsymbol{\gamma}. \tag{5.41}$$

Proof *The ethical loss associated with the target $\boldsymbol{\pi}$ is $\theta_{\max}-\sum_{j=1}^{v} \pi_j \theta_j$ and it must be less than or equal to the loss associated with the best target for inference $\theta_{\max}-\sum_{j=1}^{v} \pi_{\mathcal{I}}^* \theta_j$.*

Example 5.9 *For a binary response trial let $\mathbf{p}^t=(p_1, \ldots, p_v)$ and suppose that the criterion of interest is D-optimality Φ_D; then the inferentially optimal target is the balanced one. Thus, an allocation $\boldsymbol{\pi}$ is admissible with respect to $(\Phi_D; \tilde{\mathcal{E}})$ if and only if*

$$\mathbf{p}^t \boldsymbol{\pi} \geq v^{-1} \mathbf{p}^t \mathbf{1}_v=\frac{1}{v} \sum_{j=1}^{v} p_j\,,$$

namely if and only if $\boldsymbol{\pi}$ skews the allocations by favouring the treatments with success probabilities greater than the average.

5.6.2 Combined and constrained optimal targets for v treatments

Using the analytical expressions of the inferential and ethical criteria given in Section 5.6.1, it is possible to derive optimal target allocations of v treatments via the constrained and combined optimization methodologies discussed in Sections 5.4 and 5.5.

Starting with the compound approach, the definitions of the criteria Ψ_ω in (5.22) and $\tilde{\Psi}_\omega$ in (5.31) are the same, i.e.,

$$\Psi_\omega(\boldsymbol{\pi})=(1-\omega)\, \Psi_1(\boldsymbol{\pi})+\omega \Psi_2(\boldsymbol{\pi}), \tag{5.42}$$

and

$$\tilde{\Psi}_\omega(\boldsymbol{\pi})=\omega\left[\frac{1}{1-\Psi_2(\boldsymbol{\pi})}\right]+(1-\omega)\left[\frac{1}{1-\Psi_1(\boldsymbol{\pi})}\right]. \tag{5.43}$$

As shown previously, the ethical weight ω may be fixed a priori or could be modeled as a function of the unknown parameters $\boldsymbol{\theta}$. In the latter case, ω should be chosen so as to to deal with all the treatments symmetrically and assumed to be an increasing function of a suitable dissimilarity measure of the treatment effects (e.g., the range or the variance of $\theta_1, \ldots, \theta_v$), since it is reasonable to suppose that the more the effects of the treatments differ, the more important for the subjects is the chance of receiving the best treatment, whereas in the case of a small difference, which is more difficult to detect correctly, more emphasis is given on inferential precision. For instance, we could let $\omega=\omega(\theta_{\max}-\theta_{\min}): \mathbb{R}^+ \cup \{0\} \rightarrow [0;1)$ be a continuous and increasing function with $\omega(0)=0$ (clearly, in the case of binary trials the domain of $\omega(\cdot)$ should be suitably re-scaled).

As shown previously, if both criteria Ψ_1 and Ψ_2 are strictly convex differentiable functions, then the optimal combined target $\boldsymbol{\pi}_\omega^*$ minimizing the chosen compromise criterion is unique and can be obtained by standard differentiation techniques. For instance, assuming Ψ_ω in (5.42) then $\boldsymbol{\pi}^*_\omega$ is the solution of the set of equations

$$\omega\nabla(\Psi_2(\boldsymbol{\pi})) + (1-\omega)\nabla(\Psi_1(\boldsymbol{\pi})) = \mathbf{0}\,,$$

where $\nabla g(\cdot)$ denotes the gradient of the function $g(\cdot)$.

Example 5.10 *For binary response trials, let $\tilde{\mathcal{E}}$ in (5.40) and Φ_D be the criteria of interest. Therefore*

$$\tilde{\mathcal{E}}(\boldsymbol{\pi}^*_{\mathcal{E}}) = q_{\min} \quad \textit{and} \quad \Phi_D(\boldsymbol{\pi}^*_{\mathcal{I}}) = 2^v \prod_{j=1}^{v} p_j q_j\,,$$

and assuming the compound criterion (5.43), from (5.34) it follows that

$$\begin{aligned}\tilde{\Psi}_\omega(\boldsymbol{\pi}) &= \omega\left[\frac{\tilde{\mathcal{E}}(\boldsymbol{\pi})}{q_{min}}\right] + (1-\omega)\left[\frac{\Phi_D(\boldsymbol{\pi})}{2^v\prod_{j=1}^{v} p_j q_j}\right] \\ &= \omega\sum_{j=1}^{v}\pi_j\left(\frac{q_j}{q_{min}}\right) + (1-\omega)\left[2^v\prod_{j=1}^{v}\pi_j\right]^{-1}.\end{aligned} \tag{5.44}$$

Thus the optimal combined target $\boldsymbol{\pi}^*_\omega$ is the solution of the set of equations:

$$\begin{cases} \frac{1}{\pi_1} - \frac{1}{\pi_2} = \frac{\omega}{1-\omega}\left(\frac{q_1-q_2}{q_{\min}}\right) 2^v \prod_{j=1}^{v}\pi_j, \\ \vdots \\ \frac{1}{\pi_1} - \frac{1}{\pi_v} = \frac{\omega}{1-\omega}\left(\frac{q_1-q_v}{q_{\min}}\right) 2^v \prod_{j=1}^{v}\pi_j. \end{cases} \tag{5.45}$$

Adopting a constrained approach, by (5.15) the problem lies in finding the allocation $\boldsymbol{\pi}^*_C$ that minimizes the (ethical) criterion Ψ_2 for a chosen threshold C of maximum loss of (inferential) efficiency expressed by criterion Ψ_1. When Ψ_1 and Ψ_2 are strictly convex differentiable functions of $\boldsymbol{\pi}$, this is a convex optimization problem and therefore the Karush–Kuhn–Tucker (KKT) first order conditions are necessary and sufficient (see for instance Boyd and Vandenberghe (2004)) to guarantee a unique optimal solution $\boldsymbol{\pi}^*_C$ obtained by solving

$$\nabla(\Psi_2(\boldsymbol{\pi}^*_C)) + \kappa\nabla(\Psi_1(\boldsymbol{\pi}^*_C)) = \mathbf{0}\,,$$

where $\kappa \geq 0$ is the KKT multiplier and

$$\kappa\left[\Psi_1(\boldsymbol{\pi}^*_C) - C\right] = 0.$$

Example 5.11 *For binary response trials, Sverdlov and Rosenberger (2013a) have proposed a generalization of the target π^*_R in (5.12) to the case of several treatments. Let Φ_{A_L} in (5.37) and $\tilde{\mathcal{E}}$ in (5.40) be the criteria of interest, so that the goal is to* *minimize the total expected number of failures subject to a restriction on the trace of* $\mathbf{L}^t\mathbf{M}^{-1}(\boldsymbol{\theta} \mid \boldsymbol{\pi})\mathbf{L}$ *given by (5.38). The optimization problem becomes*

$$\begin{cases} \textit{minimize} & \boldsymbol{\pi}^t\mathbf{q}, \\ \textit{subject to} & n^{-1}\left[(v-1)\frac{p_1q_1}{\pi_1} + \sum_{j=2}^{v}\frac{p_jq_j}{\pi_j}\right] = \tilde{C}. \end{cases} \tag{5.46}$$

Therefore, the unique optimal constrained target $\boldsymbol{\pi}_C^* = (\pi_{C1}^*, \ldots, \pi_{Cv}^*)^t$ *solving (5.46) is given by*

$$\pi_{C1}^* = \frac{\sqrt{p_1(v-1)}}{\sqrt{p_1(v-1)} + \sum_{j=2}^{v}\sqrt{p_j}},$$

$$\pi_{Cl}^* = \frac{\sqrt{p_l}}{\sqrt{p_1(v-1)} + \sum_{j=2}^{v}\sqrt{p_j}}, \qquad l = 2, \ldots, v.$$

For $v = 3$ *treatments with* $\mathbf{p} = (0.35, 0.65, 0.01)^t$*, the ensuing target is* $\boldsymbol{\pi}_C^* = (0.48, 0.46, 0.06)^t$*. Adopting this constrained optimal allocation the majority of subjects (around 50%) are assigned to treatment* T_1*, even if* T_2 *is extremely more efficient. This is clearly due to the choice of the inferential criterion, since all the contrasts are evaluated with respect to* T_1*, so that the importance of the first treatment will be overestimated and this conflicts with the ethical goal. At the same time, the proportion of assignments to* T_3 *is very small, due to the joint effect of both ethical and inferential skewing.*

6

Randomization procedures that depend on the covariates

6.1 Introduction

Real life experiments, and in particular clinical trials, usually involve additional information on the experimental units, in the form of a set of covariates, e.g., important prognostic factors for patients. Taking these covariates into account is of primary importance for a correct inference, and it must be a fundamental concern from a design perspective in sequential experiments as well. The literature on adaptive randomization has been focusing the attention on this issue; see for instance Rosenberger and Lachin (2002), Hu and Rosenberger (2006), Rosenberger and Sverdlov (2008) and Shao et al. (2010).

Zelen (1974), Taves (1974) and other pioneering authors introduced adaptive designs adjusted for covariates in order to ensure approximate balance between the treatment arms in a set of pre-specified categorical covariates. These methods modify the allocation probabilities at each step according to previous assignments and the characteristics of previous subjects, as well as those of the current one, with the aim of reducing possible sources of heterogeneity and related biases. In general, these procedures – known as minimization and stratified randomization methods – have an intuitive appeal, and are fairly simple to implement. These designs have become very popular and are widely used in clinical practice to this day.

The minimization methods, usually associated to the names of Pocock and Simon (1975), were originally introduced by Taves (1974) in a deterministic version. They are aimed at achieving the so-called *marginal balance*, namely the balance between the treatment arms within each level of every covariate. They do not assume a formal statistical model and the allocation rule does not depend on the observed responses. Since deterministic procedures are subject to several types of bias, the original method was later modified introducing a random component in the allocations by means of a biased coin (Pocock and Simon, 1975; Barbachano et al., 2008) or an urn mechanism (Wei, 1978b), of the types seen in the previous chapters. Moreover, since in practice some covariates may have a greater impact on the outcome than others, minimization methods have been subsequently modified in order to differentiate the role of the covariates and, consequently, the need for balance at their various levels (Signorini et al., 1993; Heritier et al., 2005).

The stratified randomization methods, on the other hand, aim to achieve the so-called *joint balance*, or *balance within strata*, i.e., balance within each combination of the covariate levels. They generate a separate randomization sequence within each covariate profile, usually based on Complete Randomization or Permuted Block Designs (Zelen, 1974; Efron, 1980; Kaiser, 2012). However, complete randomization may induce strongly unbalanced groups, and this is particularly critical when the number of subjects recruited in each stratum is small, i.e., in the case of small sample trials or when the number of strata is high. Also, Permuted Block Designs with small size blocks tend to be highly predictable due to the deterministic component inherent in them, as seen in Chapter 2.

Simulation studies performed by several authors (see for instance Pocock and Simon (1975), Begg and Iglewicz (1980), Zielhuis et al. (1990), Atkinson (1999) and Atkinson (2002)) have shown that both minimization methods and stratified randomization can induce a significant loss of inferential precision as the number of chosen covariates and/or their levels grows. A better understanding of the theoretical properties of these methods is not available and might be helpful.

A different approach is to assume a statistical model and apply the methodology of Optimal Design theory: some covariate-adaptive randomization rules have been proposed that minimize the variance of the estimated difference between the treatment effects. In particular, those suggested by Begg and Iglewicz (1980), Atkinson (1982) and Smith (1984a) achieve balance sequentially when the model is a linear homoscedastic one without treatment/covariate interaction. These designs are better justified from a mathematical perspective and can be applied with qualitative and/or quantitative covariates, but their implementation is fairly complex, since numerical optimization algorithms are required. Moreover, their efficiency is strongly related to the model assumptions, in particular the homoscedasticity of the outcomes, which somewhat limits their applicability.

Yet another different viewpoint is the Covariate-Adjusted Response-Adaptive (CARA) randomization (Rosenberger et al., 2001b; Hu and Rosenberger, 2006; Zhang et al., 2007b). These are allocation methods that sequentially modify the treatment assignments on the basis of earlier responses, earlier allocations, past covariate profiles and the characteristics of the subject under consideration. The aim is skewing the allocations towards the superior treatment or, more in general, of converging to a desired target allocation that depends on the chosen covariates.

All the above topics are included in this chapter. Section 6.2 sets the notation and discusses the importance of balanced designs under the assumptions of a linear homoscedastic model incorporating covariates. Section 6.3 is about the sequential methods that adapt for covariates regardless of the responses, namely minimization, the procedures based on Optimal Design theory and the stratified randomization mechanisms formalized in the general class of Covariate-adaptive Biased Coin Designs by Baldi Antognini and Zagoraiou (2011); included is Hu and Hu's Covariate-adaptive allocation rule, that combines in a unique framework stratified randomization and minimization. Section 6.4 is about CARA designs. In particular, we discuss the CARA design suggested by Zhang et al. (2007b), which is an extension of the SML design of Chapter 3 to the case with covariates, the Covariate-adjusted Doubly-adaptive Biased Coin Design by Zhang and Hu (2009), namely a Doubly-adaptive BCD adjusted for covariates which at each step forces the allocations towards the target, and the Reinforced Doubly-adaptive Biased Coin design (Baldi Antognini and Zagoraiou, 2012), namely a general class of CARA procedures for categorical covariates that converges to any pre-determined allocation proportion forcing closeness to the target on the basis of the different representativeness of the covariate profiles. Section 6.5 is devoted to compound optimal designs that combine efficiency with ethical or economical gain making use of the covariates. Section 6.6 mentions some suggestions of designs for models with covariates other than the linear homoscedastic one.

To avoid cumbersome notation, in the present chapter we restrict ourselves to the case of just two treatments, but in general the definitions and results can be extended to any number $v > 2$ (see Atkinson (1982), Smith (1984a), Smith (1984b), Hu and Rosenberger (2006) and Zhang et al. (2007b)).

6.2 Inferentially optimal target allocations in the presence of covariates

In this section we discuss the optimality of balancing the treatment allocations when the statistical model is a linear homoscedastic one with covariates. The meaning of "balanced covariates" is different according to the context. In the model, the covariates may or may not be assumed to interact with the treatments and, in case of more than one covariate, may or may not be assumed to interact among themselves. These cases must be discussed separately, in order to emphasize their implications for the design.

6.2.1 Balanced designs for the linear model without treatment/covariate interactions

We suppose that for each subject entering the experiment we observe a vector $\boldsymbol{Z} = (Z_1, \ldots, Z_p)^t$ of concomitant variables, which may be categorical (blocks) or quantitative: thus we take each observed covariate to be identified either by a vector of dummies indicating its level, or by a numerical value ranging in an interval. We assume the covariates to be random, i.e., they are not under the experimenter's control but can be measured on each unit before assigning a treatment. Then the unit is allocated to one of the treatments according to a given deterministic or randomized rule and the response is observed. Conditionally on the covariates and the treatments, outcomes are assumed to be independent.

With two treatments A and B, a common model for the response is the linear homoscedastic one

$$E[Y_i] = \delta_i\mu_A + (1-\delta_i)\mu_B + \boldsymbol{h}(\boldsymbol{z}_i)^t\boldsymbol{\beta}, \qquad Var[Y_i] = \sigma^2, \qquad i \geq 1, \quad (6.1)$$

where μ_A and μ_B are the treatment effects, $\boldsymbol{z}_i$ is the vector of covariates observed on the ith unit, $\boldsymbol{h}(\cdot)$ is a known vector function which may include interactions among the covariates and $\boldsymbol{\beta}$ is a d-dimensional vector of covariate effects. We also assume the vectors $\mathbf{Z}_i$ to be iid. Note that model (6.1) does not account for treatment/covariate interactions: for each subject's profile the difference between the treatment effects is $\mu_A - \mu_B$, so that the superiority or inferiority of treatment A over B is *uniformly* constant over the covariates (the so-called hypothesis of *parallelism* of the treatment effects).

Suppose that n assignments of either treatment A or B have been made. Letting $\mathbf{Y} = (Y_1, \ldots, Y_n)^t$, $\delta^{(n)} = (\delta_1, \ldots, \delta_n)^t$, $Z^{(n)} = (\boldsymbol{Z}_1, \ldots, \boldsymbol{Z}_n)^t$ and $\mathbf{F}_n = (\boldsymbol{h}(\boldsymbol{z}_i)^t)_{n \times d}$, model (6.1) can be written as follows

$$E[\mathbf{Y}] = \mathbf{X}\boldsymbol{\gamma} = \delta^{(n)}\mu_A + \left(\mathbf{1}_n - \delta^{(n)}\right)\mu_B + \mathbf{F}_n\boldsymbol{\beta}, \quad Var[\mathbf{Y}] = \sigma^2 \mathbf{I}_n,$$

where $\mathbf{X} = \left(\delta^{(n)} : \mathbf{1}_n - \delta^{(n)} : \mathbf{F}_n\right)$ and $\boldsymbol{\gamma}^t = (\mu_A, \mu_B, \boldsymbol{\beta}^t)$ denotes the vector of unknown parameters.

Let $\hat{\gamma}_n = (\hat{\mu}_{An}, \hat{\mu}_{Bn}, \hat{\boldsymbol{\beta}}_n^t)^t$ be the Least Square estimator of $\boldsymbol{\gamma}$, then if $(\mathbf{X}^t\mathbf{X})^{-1}$ exists, the full $(2+d)$-dim normalized information matrix of the parameter vector $\boldsymbol{\gamma}$, given the covariates and the design, is

$$\mathbf{M} = \begin{pmatrix} \pi_n & 0 & n^{-1}\delta^{(n)t}\mathbf{F}_n \\ 0 & 1-\pi_n & n^{-1}\left(\mathbf{1}_n - \delta^{(n)}\right)^t \mathbf{F}_n \\ n^{-1}\mathbf{F}_n^t\delta^{(n)} & n^{-1}\mathbf{F}_n^t\left(\mathbf{1}_n - \delta^{(n)}\right) & n^{-1}\mathbf{F}_n^t\mathbf{F}_n \end{pmatrix}, \tag{6.2}$$

(see Example A.6 in Appendix A).

In the absence of treatment/covariate interaction, the covariates affect the treatment responses in the same way for all subjects. In this case it is customary to regard the vector $\boldsymbol{\beta}$ as nuisance parameter, so that the inferential interest typically lies in estimating (μ_A, μ_B) or $\mu_A - \mu_B$ as precisely as possible. Letting $\mathbf{L}^t = (\mathbf{I}_2 : \mathbf{0}_{2\times d})$, where $\mathbf{0}_{h\times d}$ denotes the $(h \times d)$-dimensional matrix of zeroes, the optimality criteria of interest are:

$$\operatorname{tr} Var[\hat{\mu}_A, \hat{\mu}_B] = n^{-1}\sigma^2 \operatorname{tr}\left(\mathbf{L}^t\mathbf{M}^{-1}\mathbf{L}\right), \tag{6.3}$$

$$\det Var[\hat{\mu}_A, \hat{\mu}_B] = n^{-1}\sigma^2 \det\left(\mathbf{L}^t\mathbf{M}^{-1}\mathbf{L}\right), \tag{6.4}$$

and

$$Var[\hat{\mu}_A - \hat{\mu}_B] = n^{-1}\sigma^2(1,-1)\mathbf{L}^t\mathbf{M}^{-1}\mathbf{L}(1,-1)^t, \tag{6.5}$$

with $\mathbf{M}^{-1}$ replaced by the Moore–Penrose generalized inverse if needed.

The *balance condition* (see equations (A.9) and (A.10) in Appendix A) is now

$$\left(2\delta^{(n)} - \mathbf{1}_n\right)^t (\mathbf{1}_n : \mathbf{F}_n) = \mathbf{0}_{1\times(d+1)}. \tag{6.6}$$

A design with this property is optimal for model (6.1) with respect to (6.3), (6.4) and (6.5). In (6.6) the quantity $\boldsymbol{b}_n^t = (2\delta^{(n)} - \mathbf{1}_n)^t(\mathbf{1}_n : \mathbf{F}_n)$ is usually called the *imbalance vector*; because its first element is equal to zero, i.e.,

$$\left(2\delta^{(n)} - \mathbf{1}_n\right)^t \mathbf{1}_n = D_n = 0,$$

the two treatments are *globally* equireplicated.

6.2.2 Marginal balance versus joint balance

In order to clarify the different types of balances that can arise in the presence of covariates and their properties, from now on for simplicity we take into account the case of two covariates $\boldsymbol{Z} = (T, W)$.

When both covariates are quantitative and in the absence of interactions, condition $(2\delta^{(n)} - \mathbf{1}_n)^t \mathbf{F}_n = \mathbf{0}_{1\times d}$ means the equality of the sums of the covariates in the two arms, so (6.6) ensures that for each covariate the averages in the treatment arms are the same. In the presence of interactions, it also implies the equality of the covariances in the two arms.

As regards categorical covariates, suppose that T is categorized into $(J+1)$ levels $t_0, t_1, \ldots, t_J$, so T can be represented by a J-dimensional vector $\mathbb{T}$ of dummy variables; similarly, let $w_0, w_1, \ldots, w_L$ be the levels of W, which can be represented by a L-dimensional vector $\mathbb{W}$ of dummies. Under this parametrization t_0 and w_0 are the so-called reference categories, namely every effect must be interpreted with respect to the (null) reference effect of t_0 and w_0. In this setting each stratum will be denoted by (j, l), while we use t_j and w_l for the two margins to avoid ambiguities (for $j = 0, \ldots, J$ and $l = 0, \ldots, L$).

Assume either

$$\boldsymbol{h}(\boldsymbol{z})^t = (\mathbb{T}^t, \mathbb{W}^t)$$

or

$$\boldsymbol{h}(\boldsymbol{z})^t = (\mathbb{T}^t, \mathbb{W}^t, \mathbb{T}^t \otimes \mathbb{W}^t), \tag{6.7}$$

on the basis of the absence or presence of all the interactions among covariates, respectively. After n assignments, let $D_n(t_j)$ be the difference between the number of subjects assigned to A and those assigned to B within the level t_j of T ($j = 0, \ldots, J$) and, similarly, let $D_n(w_l)$ represent the imbalance between the two arms at the category w_l of W ($l = 0, \ldots, L$). Moreover, let $D_n(j, l)$ be the imbalance within the stratum (j, l) ($j = 0, \ldots, J$ and $l = 0, \ldots, L$). In the absence of interactions, condition (6.6) becomes

$$\mathbf{b}_n^t = (D_n, D_n(t_1), \ldots, D_n(t_J), D_n(w_1), \ldots, D_n(w_L)) = \mathbf{0}_{1\times(J+L+1)},$$

stating that A and B are equally replicated at every level of each covariate, namely the so-called *marginal balance*. On the other hand, under (6.7) the imbalance vector is

$$\mathbf{b}_n^t = (D_n, D_n(t_1), \ldots, D_n(t_J), D_n(w_1), \ldots, D_n(w_L), D_n(1,1), \ldots, D_n(J, L))$$

and thus (6.6) means that the two treatments are equireplicated also within every stratum, i.e., the *joint balance*, which implies the marginal one.

Clearly, when the model is not full, then $\boldsymbol{b}_n$ contains all the imbalance terms corresponding to the interactions that have been included. The notation and the interpretation are similar if one of the covariates is quantitative and the other is categorical.

Inferential criteria (6.3) and (6.4) can be rewritten, respectively, as

$$\mathrm{tr}Var\left[\hat{\mu}_A, \hat{\mu}_B\right] = \frac{\sigma^2}{n}\left(1 - \frac{L_n}{n}\right)^{-1} \tag{6.8}$$

and

$$\det Var\left[\hat{\mu}_A, \hat{\mu}_B\right] = \frac{4\sigma^4}{n\left(n - \mathbf{1}_n^t \mathbf{F}_n (\mathbf{F}_n^t \mathbf{F}_n)^{-1} \mathbf{F}_n^t \mathbf{1}_n\right)} \left(1 - \frac{L_n}{n}\right)^{-1}, \tag{6.9}$$

where the only term that depends on the design is

$$L_n = \boldsymbol{b}_n^t \begin{pmatrix} n & \mathbf{1}_n^t \mathbf{F}_n \\ \mathbf{F}_n^t \mathbf{1}_n & \mathbf{F}_n^t \mathbf{F}_n \end{pmatrix}^{-1} \boldsymbol{b}_n, \tag{6.10}$$

which measures the loss of precision associated with an experiment involving n statistical units (see Section 2.3.1 in Chapter 2).

From (6.8) and (6.9), it is easy to see that both criteria have the same standardized version given by $1 - n^{-1}L_n$, namely the inferential efficiency depends on the allocations and the covariates and is maximized if (6.6) holds true.

As shown in Baldi Antognini and Zagoraiou (2011), assuming model (6.1) with $\boldsymbol{h}(\boldsymbol{z})$ as in (6.7), the loss can be rewritten as follows

$$L_n = \sum_{j=0}^{J} \sum_{l=0}^{L} \frac{D_n^2(j,l)}{N_n(j,l)}, \tag{6.11}$$

where $N_n(j,l)$ denotes the number of subjects within stratum (j,l) after n assignments ($j = 0, \ldots, J$; $l = 0, \ldots, L$).

As mentioned previously, several designs have been suggested in the literature aimed at achieving marginal balance between the treatments. However, in the presence of interactions among covariates, balancing just the margins can induce a critical loss of precision, which may also be amplified by the random nature of the covariates, as the following example shows.

Example 6.1 *Assume model (6.1) with $\boldsymbol{Z} = (T, W)$ binary covariates potentially interacting. If the design is marginally – but not jointly – balanced, then $\mathbf{b}_n^t = (0, 0, 0, D_n(1,1))$ (with $D_n(1,1) \neq 0$) and thus*

$$L_n = D_n^2(1,1) \sum_{j,l=0}^{1} N_n(j,l)^{-1}.$$

Note that $|D_n(j,l)|$ is constant at each stratum, since the design is marginally balanced; moreover $1 \leq |D_n(j,l)| \leq \min_{jl} N_n(j,l)$ and therefore $L_n \leq 4 \min_{jl} N_n(j,l)$. Setting for instance $n = 100$ and $D_{100}(1,1) = 10$, if $N_{100}(0,0) = N_{100}(1,0) = N_{100}(0,1) = 30$, then $L_{100}/100 = 0.2$, while if $N_{100}(0,0) = N_{100}(1,0) = N_{100}(0,1) = N_{100}(1,1) = 25$ and $D_{100}(1,1) = 23$, then the loss of efficiency is $L_{100}/100 = 0.846$.

Thus, within-strata imbalance may decrease the inferential precision dramatically, due to interactions among covariates and the random arrival of units in the strata. With interactions among covariates there are several marginally unbalanced designs that perform better than marginally balanced ones (see for instance Baldi Antognini and Zagoraiou (2011)).

6.2.3 Balanced designs for the linear model with treatment/covariate interactions

The assumption that each treatment affects in the same way all the subjects independently of their characteristics leads, however, to a very simplified scenario which strongly restricts its applicability in statistical practice. Thus, instead of (6.1), a more realistic model that accounts for the general situation of treatment/covariate interactions is the linear homoscedastic model in the form

$$E[Y_i] = \delta_i\,\mu_A + (1-\delta_i)\,\mu_B + \boldsymbol{h}(\boldsymbol{z}_i)^t\,(\delta_i\boldsymbol{\beta}_A + (1-\delta_i)\boldsymbol{\beta}_B) \qquad i \geq 1, \quad (6.12)$$

where now $\boldsymbol{\beta}_A$ and $\boldsymbol{\beta}_B$ are d-dim vectors of possibly different regression parameters. Under (6.12), the vector of unknown model parameters is now $\boldsymbol{\gamma} = (\mu_A, \mu_B, \boldsymbol{\beta}_A^t, \boldsymbol{\beta}_B^t)^t$ and the corresponding $(2+2d)$-dim information matrix is

$$\mathbf{M} = \begin{pmatrix} \pi_n & 0 & n^{-1}\delta^{(n)t}\mathbf{F}_n & \mathbf{0}_{1\times d} \\ 0 & 1-\pi_n & \mathbf{0}_{1\times d} & n^{-1}(\mathbf{1}_n - \delta^{(n)})^t\mathbf{F}_n \\ n^{-1}\mathbf{F}_n^t\delta^{(n)} & \mathbf{0}_{d\times 1} & n^{-1}\mathbf{F}_n^t\tilde{\boldsymbol{\Delta}}\mathbf{F}_n & \mathbf{0}_{d\times d} \\ \mathbf{0}_{d\times 1} & n^{-1}\mathbf{F}_n^t(\mathbf{1}_n - \delta^{(n)}) & \mathbf{0}_{d\times d} & n^{-1}\mathbf{F}_n^t(\mathbf{I}_n - \tilde{\boldsymbol{\Delta}})\mathbf{F}_n \end{pmatrix}, \quad (6.13)$$

with $\tilde{\boldsymbol{\Delta}} = diag\left(\delta^{(n)}\right)$.

Assuming model (6.12), the entire parameter vector $\boldsymbol{\gamma}^t = (\mu_A, \mu_B, \boldsymbol{\beta}_A^t, \boldsymbol{\beta}_B^t)$ is now of interest, since the relative performance of the treatments depends on the subject's covariates. Indeed, for any given profile $\boldsymbol{z}$ the difference between the treatment effects is (for all $i \geq 1$)

$$\begin{aligned} \zeta(\boldsymbol{z}) &= E[Y_i \mid \delta_i = 1, \boldsymbol{Z}_i = \boldsymbol{z}] - E[Y_i \mid \delta_i = 0, \boldsymbol{Z}_i = \boldsymbol{z}] \\ &= \mu_A - \ \mu_B + \boldsymbol{h}(\boldsymbol{z})^t\,(\boldsymbol{\beta}_A - \boldsymbol{\beta}_B)\,. \end{aligned} \quad (6.14)$$

Let $\hat{\boldsymbol{\gamma}}_n^t = (\hat{\mu}_{An}, \hat{\mu}_{Bn}, \hat{\boldsymbol{\beta}}_{An}^t, \hat{\boldsymbol{\beta}}_{Bn}^t)$ be the OLS estimator of the unknown model parameters after n assignments, and $\mathbf{D}^t = (\mathbf{0}_{2d\times 2} : \mathbf{I}_{2d})$. Some inferential criteria of interest are now

$$\det Var[\hat{\boldsymbol{\gamma}}_n] = \det\left(\frac{\sigma^2}{n}\mathbf{M}^{-1}\right), \quad (6.15)$$

$$\det Var\left[\hat{\boldsymbol{\beta}}_A^t, \hat{\boldsymbol{\beta}}_B^t\right] = \det\left(\frac{\sigma^2}{n}\mathbf{D}^t\mathbf{M}^{-1}\mathbf{D}\right), \quad (6.16)$$

$$\mathrm{tr}\, Var\left[\hat{\boldsymbol{\gamma}}_n\right] = \mathrm{tr}\left(\frac{\sigma^2}{n}\mathbf{M}^{-1}\right), \quad (6.17)$$

$$\mathrm{tr}\, Var\left[\hat{\boldsymbol{\beta}}_A^t, \hat{\boldsymbol{\beta}}_B^t\right] = \mathrm{tr}\left(\frac{\sigma^2}{n}\mathbf{D}^t\mathbf{M}^{-1}\mathbf{D}\right) \quad (6.18)$$

where $\mathbf{M}$ is now (6.13).

For model (6.12) the *balance condition* of Appendix A, Example A.7, becomes

$$\left(2\delta^{(n)} - \mathbf{1}_n\right)^t (\mathbf{1}_n : \mathbf{F}_n) = \mathbf{0}_{1\times(d+1)} \quad (6.19)$$

$$\mathbf{F}_n^t(2\tilde{\boldsymbol{\Delta}} - \mathbf{I}_n)\mathbf{F}_n = \mathbf{0}_{d\times d} \quad (6.20)$$

and is optimal for model (6.12) with respect to criteria (6.15) through (6.18).

In the absence of interactions, i.e., $\boldsymbol{h}(\boldsymbol{z})^t = (t, w)$, in addition to the equality of the averages in the treatment arms implied by (6.19), (6.20) implies that

$$\sum_{i=1}^{n} \delta_i t_i^2 = \sum_{i=1}^{n} (1-\delta_i) t_i^2, \qquad \sum_{i=1}^{n} \delta_i w_i^2 = \sum_{i=1}^{n} (1-\delta_i) w_i^2$$
$$\text{and} \quad \sum_{i=1}^{n} \delta_i t_i w_i = \sum_{i=1}^{n} (1-\delta_i) t_i w_i\,, \tag{6.21}$$

namely for each covariate their variances in the two arms are the same, as well as the covariances. If $\boldsymbol{h}(\boldsymbol{z})^t = (t, w, t \cdot w)$, in addition to (6.21), (6.20) also implies that

$$\sum_{i=1}^{n} \delta_i t_i^2 w_i = \sum_{i=1}^{n} (1-\delta_i) t_i^2 w_i, \qquad \sum_{i=1}^{n} \delta_i t_i w_i^2 = \sum_{i=1}^{n} (1-\delta_i) t_i w_i^2$$
$$\text{and} \quad \sum_{i=1}^{n} \delta_i t_i^2 w_i^2 = \sum_{i=1}^{n} (1-\delta_i) t_i^2 w_i^2\,.$$

Let the categorical covariates of interest be $\boldsymbol{Z} = (T, W)^t$, and let $\pi_n(j, l)$ be the proportion of allocations to treatment A within stratum (j, l) after n assignments ($j = 0, \ldots, J$ and $l = 0, \ldots, L$). Assuming model (6.12) with (6.7), Baldi Antognini and Zagoraiou (2012) have shown that criteria (6.15) through (6.18) can be simplified as follows:

$$\det\left(\frac{\sigma^2}{n}\mathbf{M}^{-1}\right) = \frac{\sigma^{4+4p}}{\prod_{j=0}^{J}\prod_{l=0}^{L} \pi_n(j,l)[1-\pi_n(j,l)]N_n(j,l)^2}, \tag{6.22}$$

$$\det\left(\frac{\sigma^2}{n}\mathbf{D}^t\mathbf{M}^{-1}\mathbf{D}\right) = \frac{n^2\pi_n(1-\pi_n)\sigma^{4p}}{\prod_{j=0}^{J}\prod_{l=0}^{L} \pi_n(j,l)[1-\pi_n(j,l)]N_n(j,l)^2}, \tag{6.23}$$

$$\begin{aligned}\operatorname{tr}\left(\frac{\sigma^2}{n}\mathbf{M}^{-1}\right) &= \sigma^2 \times \Big[\sum_{j=1}^{J}\sum_{l=1}^{L} \frac{1}{N_n(j,l)\pi_n(j,l)[1-\pi_n(j,l)]} + \\ &+ \sum_{j=1}^{J} \frac{L+1}{N_n(j,0)\pi_n(j,0)[1-\pi_n(j,0)]} + \sum_{l=1}^{L} \frac{J+1}{N_n(0,l)\pi_n(0,l)[1-\pi_n(0,l)]} + \\ &+ \frac{(J+1)\times(L+1)}{N_n(0,0)\pi_n(0,0)[1-\pi_n(0,0)]}\Big]\end{aligned} \tag{6.24}$$

and

$$\operatorname{tr}\left(\frac{\sigma^2}{n}\mathbf{D}^t\mathbf{M}^{-1}\mathbf{D}\right) = \operatorname{tr}\left(\frac{\sigma^2}{n}\mathbf{M}^{-1}\right) - \frac{\sigma^2}{N_n(0,0)\pi_n(0,0)[1-\pi_n(0,0)]}. \tag{6.25}$$

Criteria (6.22) through (6.25) are minimized by the jointly balanced design, which is still optimal in the absence of interactions among covariates, independently of the presence or absence of treatment/covariate interactions.

6.3 Covariate-adaptive randomization

The previous section deals with the optimality of balanced covariates for fixed sample size. The present section discusses adaptive designs suggested for achieving some form of balance sequentially with respect to a given set of covariates of interest.

6.3.1 Pocock and Simon's minimization methods

The minimization methods proposed by Taves (1974) and analyzed in depth by Pocock and Simon (1975) are very popular methodologies in the clinical practice. They are covariate-adaptive randomization procedures aimed at achieving marginal balance. These methods depend in general on the definition of a measure of overall imbalance among the assignments, which summarizes the imbalances between the treatment groups for each level of each factor: at each step the imbalance that would occur if that subject were allocated to either treatment is calculated; then the assignment is directed (deterministically, or in a randomized way) to the treatment that minimizes the given measure of overall imbalance.

In the case of two covariates $\boldsymbol{Z} = (T, W)$, minimization methods work as follows. Let $\Im_n = \sigma\{\boldsymbol{Z}_1, \ldots, \boldsymbol{Z}_n; \delta_1, \ldots, \delta_n\}$ be the sequence of assignments and covariates up to n; when the covariate profile $\boldsymbol{z}_{n+1} = (t_j, w_l)$ of the $(n+1)$st subject is recorded, the effect on the overall imbalance of assigning treatment A or B can be measured, respectively, by $|D_n(t_j) + 1| + |D_n(w_l) + 1|$ and $|D_n(t_j) - 1| + |D_n(w_l) - 1|$. Thus, letting

$$\widetilde{D}_n = |D_n(t_j) + 1| - |D_n(t_j) - 1| + |D_n(w_l) + 1| - |D_n(w_l) - 1| \qquad (6.26)$$

be the measure of overall imbalance, this subject will be allocated to treatment A with probability

$$\Pr(\delta_{n+1} = 1 \mid \Im_n, \boldsymbol{Z}_{n+1} = (j, l)) = \begin{cases} p & \widetilde{D}_n < 0 \\ \frac{1}{2} & \widetilde{D}_n = 0\,, \\ 1-p & \widetilde{D}_n > 0 \end{cases} \qquad n \geq 1, \qquad (6.27)$$

with $p \in [1/2; 1]$. This rule is usually referred to as the *range method*, since the imbalance at each level of every covariate is measured by the range between the allocations of the two arms, i.e., $|D_n(\cdot)|$. The choice $p = 1$ corresponds to Taves' minimization method, while Pocock and Simon (1975) have studied the case $p = 3/4$ (see also Wei (1978b)).

This is a design that treats all the covariates in the same way; rule (6.27) can be simply rewritten as:

$$\Pr(\delta_{n+1} = 1 \mid \Im_n, \boldsymbol{Z}_{n+1} = (j, l)) = \begin{cases} p & \mathrm{sgn} D_n(t_j) + \mathrm{sgn} D_n(w_l) < 0, \\ \frac{1}{2} & \mathrm{sgn} D_n(t_j) + \mathrm{sgn} D_n(w_l) = 0, \\ 1-p & \mathrm{sgn} D_n(t_j) + \mathrm{sgn} D_n(w_l) > 0. \end{cases} \qquad (6.28)$$

In the case of several covariates the overall imbalance $\widetilde{D}_n$ is proportional to the sum of the signs of all the marginal imbalances of the current stratum, so that the allocation of A is forced if the number of covariates with negative imbalance is greater than the one with positive imbalance, and vice versa for B.

There follows from (6.28) that, at each step:

- the allocation depends only on the sign of the overall measure of imbalance and not on its magnitude;
- the overall measure of imbalance depends only on the signs of the current marginal imbalances related to the subject's stratum.

Example 6.2 *In order to explore how minimization methods work in practice and their drawbacks, consider now a hypothetical trial where the covariates are Cholesterol Level (with levels High and Low) and Gender (Male and Female). Suppose that the first 100 subjects have been already randomized according to either of the two scenarios illustrated in Table 6.1.*

TABLE 6.1: Minimization methods: two different scenarios.

	Scenario 1			Scenario 2		
	Male	Female	$D_{100}(\cdot)$	Male	Female	$D_{100}(\cdot)$
High CL	15 (8A; 7B)	25 (13A; 12B)	2	15 (12A; 3B)	25 (20A; 5B)	24
Low CL	10 (4A; 6B)	50 (25A; 25B)	-2	10 (0A; 10B)	50 (29A; 21B)	-2
$D_{100}(\cdot)$	-1	1	0	-1	23	22

Under Scenario 1, the two treatments are equally replicated since $D_{100} = 0$; moreover, the two arms are balanced for the categories of Gender (note that there is an odd number of both males and females), and there is only a minimum imbalance for the categories of Cholesterol Level (CL). Thus, if the 101th subject accrued into the trial is male (M) with a high cholesterol level (H), then $sgnD_{100}(M) = -1$ and $sgnD_{100}(H) = 1$, so he will be randomized to the two treatments with equal probabilities. Complete randomization will also be used if the 101th subject is female with a low level of cholesterol; whereas, in the case of a male with low cholesterol level (or female with high cholesterol level), the allocation will be forced to treatment A (respectively, B) with probability $p \geq 1/2$ (see Table 6.2). However, for each subject's profile the allocation probabilities are exactly the same also under Scenario 2, although the categories female and high cholesterol level are strongly unbalanced and treatment A is globally over represented with $D_{100} = 22$.

TABLE 6.2: Allocation probabilities to treatment A of subject 101 under the range method.

	Male	Female
High CL	0.5	$1-p$
Low CL	p	0.5

As shown by the example above, the range method is insensitive to the magnitude of the observed marginal imbalances; to overcome this drawback, Pocock and Simon (1975) have discussed the possibility of assuming different measures of imbalance at each level of every covariate, instead of the range. In particular, the so-called *variance method* consists in assuming the variance of the numbers of allocations of the two treatments as a measure of marginal imbalance, so that $|D_n(t_j)|$ and $|D_n(w_l)|$ will be replaced by $[D_n(t_j)/2]^2$ and $[D_n(w_l)/2]^2$, respectively; however, since $(x+1)^2-(x-1)^2=4x$ for any integer x, instead of (6.26) the overall measure of imbalance now becomes $\widetilde{D}_n = D_n(t_j)+D_n(w_l)$, so that under the variance method the $(n+1)$th subject is assigned to treatment A with probability:

$$\Pr\left(\delta_{n+1}=1 \mid \Im_n, \boldsymbol{Z}_{n+1}=(j,l)\right) = \begin{cases} p & D_n(t_j)+D_n(w_l)<0, \\ \frac{1}{2} & D_n(t_j)+D_n(w_l)=0, \\ 1-p & D_n(t_j)+D_n(w_l)>0. \end{cases} \qquad (6.29)$$

If compared with the range method, rule (6.29) differs from (6.28) only when $D_n(t_j)>0$ and at the same time $D_n(w_l)<0$, or vice versa: in these situations the variance method is more sensitive to the magnitude of the marginal imbalances that have been actually observed.

Example 6.3 *Table 6.3 describes the probabilities of allocation to A of the* 101*st subject given by the variance method under Scenarios 1 and 2 of Table 6.1.*

TABLE 6.3: Allocation probabilities to treatment A of subject 101 under the variance method.

	Scenario 1		Scenario 2	
	Male	Female	Male	Female
High CL	$1-p$	$1-p$	$1-p$	$1-p$
Low CL	p	p	p	$1-p$

Baldi Antognini and Zagoraiou (2015) have proved that Pocock and Simon's minimization method is asymptotically balanced, both marginally and jointly; in general, theoretical results about minimization methods seem to be few and far between. Their properties have been explored extensively through simulations (Pocock and Simon, 1975; Begg and Iglewicz, 1980; Zielhuis et al., 1990; Atkinson, 1999, 2002). In particular, Begg and Iglewicz (1980) and Zielhuis et al. (1990) have shown that the variance method performs better than the range method, but the gain in terms of inferential efficiency is moderate. Furthermore, the variance method could be inefficient due to the fact that, at each step, the allocation probability still depends only on the sign of the overall imbalance that has been currently observed and not on its magnitude. In the same spirit of the Adjustable BCD discussed in Section 2.4.2, a generalization of minimization procedures that accounts for different degrees of imbalance at each factor levels is

$$\Pr\left(\delta_{n+1}=1 \mid \Im_n, \boldsymbol{Z}_{n+1}=(j,l)\right)=F(h_T(D_n(t_j))+h_W(D_n(w_l))), \quad (6.30)$$

where $F:\mathbb{R}\to[0;1]$ is a non-increasing and symmetric function with

$$F(-x)=1-F(x), \qquad \text{for all } x\in\mathbb{R}$$

and $h_T, h_W:\mathbb{Z}\to\mathbb{R}$ are increasing functions such that

$$h_T(x)=-h_T(-x) \quad \text{and} \quad h_W(x)=-h_W(-x), \qquad \forall x\in\mathbb{Z}.$$

Rule (6.30) makes allowances for a different need for balance among the factors under consideration, in order to force the balance for the covariate or covariates that have a more prominent impact on the outcome than the others. For instance, a very simple choice consists in assuming h_T and h_W linear functions, which corresponds to assigning suitable weights to the covariates according to their importance, as we shall show in Section 6.3.4. The weights assigned to the different covariates can be chosen to correspond to the intensity of their relationship with the outcome or to their importance in response prediction. These weights may evolve adaptively and they can be estimated step by step through the available information; note that in this case the observed responses are also included in the estimation process, so that the ensuing procedure becomes a CARA design (see Section 6.4).

6.3.2 Covariate-adaptive procedures based on Optimal Design theory

Both stratified randomization procedures and minimization methods were introduced without any formal criterion of optimal inference. Being very intuitive and simple methods that do not require formulating a statistical model, they are easy to apply in practice. An alternative approach to minimization is given by the covariate-adaptive rules based on the theory of Optimal Designs (Begg and Iglewicz, 1980; Atkinson, 1982; Smith, 1984a,b; Atkinson, 2002). Adopting the linear homoscedastic model (6.1), Atkinson (1982) and Smith (1984a) have proposed procedures aimed at balancing the allocations across the covariates in order to minimize the variance of the estimated difference between the treatment effects (for a simplified version see also Begg and Iglewicz (1980)). These methods are more rigorous from a mathematical perspective and are also quite general, since they deal with any number of treatments and any type of covariates, but they are computationally expensive.

In particular, assuming the D-optimality criterion (see Appendix A) Atkinson (1982) introduced his D_A-BCD in order to minimize (6.4) sequentially. As shown previously, it corresponds to minimizing (6.10) and therefore the D_A-BCD can be generalized to account for covariates (see also Smith (1984b)) by assigning the $(n+1)$th subject to treatment A with probability

$$\Pr(\delta_{n+1}=1 \mid \Im_n, \boldsymbol{Z}_{n+1}=\boldsymbol{z}_{n+1}) =$$
$$= \frac{[1-(1;\boldsymbol{h}(\boldsymbol{z}_{n+1})^t)(\mathbb{F}_n^t\mathbb{F}_n)^{-1}\boldsymbol{b}_n]^2}{[1-(1;\boldsymbol{h}(\boldsymbol{z}_{n+1})^t)(\mathbb{F}_n^t\mathbb{F}_n)^{-1}\boldsymbol{b}_n]^2+[1+(1;\boldsymbol{h}(\boldsymbol{z}_{n+1})^t)(\mathbb{F}_n^t\mathbb{F}_n)^{-1}\boldsymbol{b}_n]^2}, \tag{6.31}$$

where $\mathbb{F}_n = (\mathbf{1}_n : \mathbf{F}_n)$ for brevity. This procedure can be naturally extended to the case of several treatments substituting criterion (6.4) with $\det(\mathbf{L}^t\mathbf{M}^{-1}\mathbf{L})$, where $\mathbf{L}$ is the matrix that specifies the contrasts of interest between the treatment effects (see Section 2.6 and Appendix A).

Assuming that the covariate distribution is known a priori and using the approximation $\mathbb{F}_n^t\mathbb{F}_n \simeq n\mathbb{Q}$ with $\mathbb{Q} = \lim_{n\to\infty} n^{-1}\mathbb{F}_n^t\mathbb{F}_n$ non-singular, Smith (1984a) has generalized Atkinson's idea by the following allocation rule

$$\Pr(\delta_{n+1}=1 \mid \Im_n, \boldsymbol{Z}_{n+1}=\boldsymbol{z}_{n+1}) = \psi(n^{-1}\boldsymbol{h}(\boldsymbol{z}_{n+1})^t\mathbb{Q}^{-1}\boldsymbol{b}_n), \tag{6.32}$$

where $\psi : [-1,1] \to [0,1]$ is a non-increasing function such that $\psi(-x) = 1-\psi(x)$ for all $x \in [-1;1]$.

For the linear model (6.1) with potentially interacting categorical covariates, Atkinson's D_A-BCD and Smith's procedures become stratified randomization methods. Indeed, assuming (6.7), then

$$(1;\boldsymbol{h}(\boldsymbol{z}_{n+1})^t)(\mathbb{F}_n^t\mathbb{F}_n)^{-1}\boldsymbol{b}_n = \frac{D_n(j,l)}{N_n(j,l)},$$

so that the D_A-BCD in (6.31) simplifies to

$$\Pr(\delta_{n+1}=1 \mid \Im_n, \boldsymbol{Z}_{n+1}=(j,l)) = \frac{\left(1-\frac{D_n(j,l)}{N_n(j,l)}\right)^2}{\left(1-\frac{D_n(j,l)}{N_n(j,l)}\right)^2+\left(1+\frac{D_n(j,l)}{N_n(j,l)}\right)^2}, \tag{6.33}$$

whereas Smith's allocation rule (6.32) becomes

$$\Pr(\delta_{n+1}=1 \mid \Im_n, \boldsymbol{Z}_{n+1}=\boldsymbol{z}_{n+1}) = \psi\left(\frac{D_n(j,l)}{N_n(j,l)}\right),$$

where $N_n(j,l)$ could be approximated by np_{jl} (see the analogy with Wei's Adaptive BCD discussed in Section 2.4.3).

Within this framework, the loss of precision in (6.10) is the fundamental tool for assessing the performances of a design; however, now the loss depends on the random covariates too. Few theoretical results are known about the distribution of L_n, mainly due to Smith (1984a,b). In particular, he proved that under rule (6.32) the expected loss converges to $(d+1)/[1-4\psi'(0)]$, provided that $\psi(\cdot)$ is a twice continuously differentiable function with uniformly bounded second derivatives. Intensive simulation studies (see Begg and Iglewicz (1980), Atkinson (1982), Atkinson (1999),

Atkinson (2002) and Heritier et al. (2005)) seem to confirm that Smith's results can be extended also to Atkinson's D_A-BCD and to the procedure suggested by Begg and Iglewicz (1980). Atkinson (1982) compared his procedure with CR and Efron's coin via simulations, which seem to show that the expected loss converges to 0 for Efron's BCD, to $(d+1)$ for CR, and to $(d+1)/5$ for the D_A-BCD. Thus, excluding Efron's coin, the asymptotic precision decreases as the number of covariates, as well as their levels and interaction effects, grows.

6.3.3 The Covariate-Adaptive Biased Coin Design introduced by Baldi Antognini and Zagoraiou

As shown previously, the optimality of marginal/joint balance depends on the absence or presence of interactions among covariates and since marginal balance does not always promote efficiency, ensuring balance within every stratum could be a crucial issue. One author among others, Kaiser (2012), pointed this out through specific examples. For this reason, Baldi Antognini and Zagoraiou (2011) have introduced the *Covariate-Adaptive Biased Coin Design* (C-ABCD), which is a general class of stratified randomization sequential methods aimed at achieving the treatment balance within strata.

Let the covariates of interest be $\boldsymbol{Z} = (T, W)$, with joint pdf $\boldsymbol{p} = [p_{jl} : j = 0, \ldots, J; l = 0, \ldots, L]$, where $p_{jl} = \Pr(\boldsymbol{Z}_i = (j, l)) > 0$ and $\sum_{j=0}^{J} \sum_{l=0}^{L} p_{jl} = 1$. For any given stratum (j, l), let $F_{jl}(\cdot) : \mathbb{Z} \to [0, 1]$ be a non-increasing and symmetric function with $F_{jl}(-x) = 1 - F_{jl}(x)$ for all $x \in \mathbb{Z}$, where $F_{jl}(\cdot)$'s are called generating functions and govern the request of balance within each covariate profile. The C-ABCD assigns the $(n+1)$th subject to treatment A with probability:

$$\Pr\left(\delta_{n+1} = 1 \mid \Im_n, \boldsymbol{Z}_{n+1} = (j, l)\right) = F_{jl}(D_n(j, l)), \qquad \text{for all } (j, l). \tag{6.34}$$

Clearly, if at each stratum (j, l) we set

$$F_{jl}(x) = \begin{cases} p & x < 0 \\ \frac{1}{2} & x = 0, \\ 1 - p & x > 0 \end{cases} \tag{6.35}$$

then rule (6.34) becomes stratified randomization, where within each stratum a separate Efron's Biased Coin Design is activated (Efron, 1980).

Remark 6.1 *In the class of restricted randomization rules that ignore covariates, like the ABCD and Wei's Adaptive BCD, the whole sequence of assignments can be determined before the trial. In the case of the C-ABCD this is not feasible, and the procedure implementation goes hand in hand with the trial itself.*

Let $\boldsymbol{D}_n = [D_n(j, l) : j = 0, \ldots, J; l = 0, \ldots, L]$. The sequence of vectors $\{\boldsymbol{D}_n\}_{n \in \mathbb{N}}$ of the C-ABCD is a positive recurrent Markov chain on $\mathbb{Z}^{(J+1)\times(L+1)}$, where each component is an ergodic random walk, but at each step n only one walk is activated, the one that corresponds to the covariate profile of subject n.

Within each stratum (j, l), for any choice of $F_{jl}(\cdot)$ the sequence $\{D_n(j,l)\}_{n\in\mathbb{N}}$ is a homogeneous Markov chain on $\mathbb{Z}$ with $D_0(j,l) = 0$ and transition probabilities

$$\Pr\left(D_{n+1}(j,l) = k \mid D_n(j,l) = x\right) = \begin{cases} p_{jl}F_{jl}(x) & k = x+1, \\ 1 - p_{jl} & k = x, \\ p_{jl}F_{jl}(-x) & k = x-1. \end{cases}$$

The chain is positive recurrent, time-reversible and aperiodic with unimodal stationary law $\xi_{jl}(\cdot)$ symmetric at 0 given by

$$\begin{aligned} \xi_{jl}(x) &= \xi_{jl}(x-1)\frac{F_{jl}(x-1)}{F_{jl}(-x)}, \qquad \text{for all } x \in \mathbb{Z} \\ \xi_{jl}(0) &= \left\{1 + 2\sum_{s=1}^{\infty}\prod_{x=1}^{s}\frac{F_{jl}(x-1)}{F_{jl}(-x)}\right\}^{-1}. \end{aligned} \tag{6.36}$$

The marginal imbalances $\{D_n(t_j)\}_{n\in\mathbb{N}}$ and $\{D_n(w_l)\}_{n\in\mathbb{N}}$, as well as the global one $\{D_n\}_{n\in\mathbb{N}}$, are also positive recurrent Markov chains on $\mathbb{Z}$, with stationary distributions that can be derived from the equilibrium equations.

For any choices of $F_{jl}(\cdot)$'s the Covariate-Adaptive Biased Coin Design is asymptotically balanced within each stratum, and also at each level of the covariates and globally:

Theorem 6.1 *Under the C-ABCD, as* $n \to \infty$

$$\frac{D_n(j,l)}{N_n(j,l)} \to 0, \quad \frac{D_n(t_j)}{N_n(t_j)} \to 0, \quad \frac{D_n(w_l)}{N_n(w_l)} \to 0 \quad \text{and} \quad \frac{D_n}{n} \to 0 \quad a.s. \tag{6.37}$$

Furthermore, the C-ABCD is high order efficient, since $\forall j = 0, \ldots, J$ and $\forall l = 0, \ldots, L$

$$D_n(j,l) = o_p(n^{1/2}),\ D_n(t_j) = o_p(n^{1/2}),\ D_n(w_l) = o_p(n^{1/2}),\ D_n = o_p(n^{1/2}) \tag{6.38}$$

and for all $\nu > 0$

$$D_n(j,l) = o_{l_1}(n^{\nu}),\ D_n(t_j) = o_{l_1}(n^{\nu}),\ D_n(w_l) = o_{l_1}(n^{\nu}),\ D_n = o_{l_1}(n^{\nu}). \tag{6.39}$$

Result (6.38) establishes that the C-ABCD converges (in probability) to balance faster than the procedures described so far, and in particular to those for which a CLT property holds, e.g., Smith's designs; whereas (6.39) establishes a high order of convergence that guarantees that the loss of efficiency L_n in (6.10) vanishes very rapidly; indeed, assuming the C-ABCD, then $L_n = o_p(1)$ independently of the number of factors taken into consideration. As a counterpart of such faster balancing properties, the C-ABCD is characterized by a small increase of selection bias; indeed, the asymptotic predictability is

$$\lim_{n\to\infty} SB_n = \frac{1}{2}\left\{\sum_{j=0}^{J}\sum_{l=0}^{L}\xi_{jl}(0)p_{jl} + 1\right\}.$$

The asymptotic excess of selection bias

$$\frac{1}{2}\sum_{j=0}^{J}\sum_{l=0}^{L}\xi_{jl}(0)p_{jl}$$

is an overall measure of asymptotic balance induced by the design over the strata.

Clearly, different choices of the generating functions for each covariate pattern meet the need for more or for less balance at different population strata. A suitable selection of $F_{jl}(\cdot)$'s is discussed in Baldi Antognini and Zagoraiou (2011), where it is shown that an interesting class of generating functions is

$$F^a(x) = \{x^a + 1\}^{-1}, \qquad x \geq 1, \tag{6.40}$$

in which the non-negative parameter $a > 0$ governs the degree of randomness: if a tends to 0 the assignment tends to be completely randomized, whereas as a grows the allocation becomes more deterministic. This class ensures a good trade-off between balance and predictability even for small samples, since the allocations are completely randomized in the case of perfect balance under an even or an odd number of steps, and the balance is forced in the other situations. The generating functions (6.40) treat each stratum in the same way, but in some circumstances there may be a need to diversify the role of some of them, since

- some patterns may have major/minor importance with respect to the others,
- strong departures from balance could induce a significant loss of precision if observed at under-represented strata, whereas their impact may be moderate if observed at populous covariate profiles.

Thus, if the covariate distribution $\boldsymbol{p}$ is known, for each stratum (j, l) a proper choice of the generating function is

$$F_{jl}(x) = \left\{x^{\frac{1-p_{jl}}{p_{jl}}} + 1\right\}^{-1}, \qquad x \geq 1; \tag{6.41}$$

when $\boldsymbol{p}$ is unknown, the generating function (6.41) could also be used substituting at each step every p_{jl} with its current estimate $\hat{p}_{njl}$; as proved by Baldi Antognini and Zagoraiou (2015), the procedure is still asymptotically balanced.

As regards finite sample comparisons, Baldi Antognini and Zagoraiou (2011) have shown via simulations that in the presence of interactions among covariates the C-ABCD yields a significant improvement in terms of inferential efficiency with respect to Pocock and Simon's procedure and Atkinson's D_A-BCD, but has slightly higher predictability with respect to the latter. Since joint implies marginal balance, the C-ABCD is still efficient even with no covariate interactions, since L_n tends to 0 as n goes to infinity, ensuring also good performances in terms of SB_n.

6.3.4 Hu and Hu's covariate-adaptive procedure

In the case of categorical covariates, Hu and Hu (2012) have introduced a class of procedures that assumes as overall measure of imbalance a weighted average of the three types of imbalances actually observed, i.e., global, marginal and within-stratum:

$$\bar{D}_n = 4\{\omega_g D_n + \omega_T D_n(t_j) + \omega_W D_n(w_l) + \omega_s D_n(j,l)\}. \tag{6.42}$$

Expression (6.42) is the measure of average imbalance after n steps for a subject belonging to the stratum (j,l) and the non-negative weight ω_g (global), ω_T and ω_W (covariate marginal) and ω_s (stratum) are such that $\omega_g + \omega_T + \omega_W + \omega_s = 1$ The allocations are randomized according to a biased coin, in such a way that each subject will be forced to the treatment which induces the smallest average imbalance.

Let the covariates of interest be $\boldsymbol{Z} = (T, W)$, this design assigns the $(n+1)$st subject to treatment A with probability

$$\Pr(\delta_{n+1} = 1 \mid \Im_n, \boldsymbol{Z}_{n+1} = (j,l)) = \begin{cases} p & \bar{D}_n < 0 \\ \frac{1}{2} & \bar{D}_n = 0 \,. \\ 1-p & \bar{D}_n > 0 \end{cases} \tag{6.43}$$

In the same spirit as Pocock and Simon (1975), $\bar{D}_n$ in (6.42) can be regarded as the difference between the weighted imbalances that would be caused if the next subject were to be assigned to treatment A or B, respectively. Clearly, if $\omega_T = \omega_W = \omega_s = 0$ rule (6.43) does not depend on the covariates and it corresponds to Efron's Biased Coin Design. When $\omega_g = \omega_s = 0$ (i.e., taking into account only the marginal imbalances), if $\omega_T = \omega_W = 0.5$ the covariates have the same relative importance and (6.43) coincides with minimization method (6.29); otherwise, the choice $\omega_T \neq \omega_W$ corresponds to a weighted version of the variance method. Moreover, if $\omega_g = \omega_T = \omega_W = 0$ then rule (6.43) becomes stratified randomization where a separate randomization mechanism based on Efron's coin is activated within each stratum, namely it becomes the special case of the C-ABCD given in (6.35).

Adopting (6.43), the sequence $\{\boldsymbol{D}_n\}_{n\in\mathbb{N}}$ is still a Markov chain and to explore the asymptotic properties of their design, Hu and Hu have obtained the conditions under which $\{\boldsymbol{D}_n\}_{n\in\mathbb{N}}$ is positive recurrent, which guarantees a fast convergence of order $O_p(1)$ for the within-stratum imbalance:

Theorem 6.2 *If the weights ω_g, ω_T, ω_W are chosen so that*

$$(JL + J + L)\omega_g + J\omega_W + L\omega_T < \frac{1}{2}, \tag{6.44}$$

then $\{\boldsymbol{D}_n\}_{n\in\mathbb{N}}$ is a positive recurrent Markov chain on $\mathbb{Z}^{(J+1)\times(L+1)}$.

Only strictly positive choices of the stratum weight ω_s satisfy Theorem 6.2. In fact, if we assume $\omega_s = 0$, then $\omega_g = 1 - \omega_T - \omega_W$ and thus condition (6.2) can be rewritten as follows

$$(JL + J + L)[1 - (\omega_W + \omega_T)] + (\omega_W + \omega_T) + \omega_W(J-1) + \omega_T(L-1) < \frac{1}{2},$$

which is clearly impossible since the LHS is always greater than 1. Thus, Theorem 6.2 does not apply to Pocock and Simon's procedure and a simulation study in Hu and Hu (2012) seems to show that under minimization method (6.29) the within-stratum imbalance $\{\boldsymbol{D}_n\}_{n\in\mathbb{N}}$ grows as n tends to infinity.

Clearly several issues still need further research. For instance, it is not clear how the marginal weights can be chosen with respect to the stratum weight: since joint balance implies marginal one and also global balance, one would expect that high values of ω_s (i.e., from Theorem 6.2, small values of ω_g, ω_T and ω_W) should be preferable, at least when the number of considered covariates is small. The relative importance of these weights, as well as the evolution of the procedure, may change as the number of chosen covariates as well as their levels grows. From the viewpoint of predictability, the theoretical properties of Hu and Hu's covariate-adaptive randomization procedure are still unclear.

6.4 Covariate-Adjusted Response-Adaptive designs

Starting from the pioneering work of Rosenberger et al. (2001b), there has been a statistical interest in the topic of Covariate-Adjusted Response-Adaptive (CARA) randomization procedures. These designs change the probabilities of allocating treatments by taking into account all the available information – namely the assignments, the outcomes and the covariates of the previous statistical units, as well as the characteristic of the current subject that will be randomized – with the aim of i) skewing the allocations towards the treatment that appears to be superior or ii) converging to a desired target allocation that depends on both the covariates and the unknown parameters of the model.

Let $\mathfrak{G}_n = \sigma\{\boldsymbol{Z}_1, \ldots, \boldsymbol{Z}_n; \delta_1, \ldots, \delta_n; Y_1 \ldots, Y_n\}$ be the sequence of covariates, assignments and responses after n steps, when the covariate profile $\boldsymbol{Z}_{n+1}$ of the $(n+1)$st subject is recorded, a CARA design is defined by

$$\Pr(\delta_{n+1} = 1 \mid \mathfrak{G}_n, \boldsymbol{Z}_{n+1}) = \varphi(\mathfrak{G}_n, \boldsymbol{Z}_{n+1}). \tag{6.45}$$

Some authors (Bandyopadhyay and Biswas, 2001; Biswas et al., 2006) have suggested CARA designs that incorporate covariate information in the randomization process, but ignore the covariates of the current subject. These methods seem to guarantee good ethical performances only asymptotically. The properties of these designs and of the estimators have been explored almost exclusively through simulations.

6.4.1 Covariate-adjusted Sequential Maximum Likelihood design

Zhang et al. (2007b) have analyzed one particular type of CARA rule that generalizes the Sequential Maximum Likelihood design (see Sections 1.9.1 and 3.3) to the presence of covariates. The assumed model is the general linear setup discussed in Section 3.2 and for any target allocation $\pi^0 \in (0;1)$ such that

- π^0 depends on both the unknown model parameters γ and the covariates, i.e., $\pi^0 = \pi^0(\gamma, z)$,
- $\pi^0(\gamma, z)$ is continuous in γ for any fixed covariate level z,

they suggest to sequentially allocate the subjects to the treatments as follows. Starting with an initial stage, where n_0 assignments of each treatment are made in order to derive a non-trivial parameter estimation $\hat{\gamma}_{2n_0}$ as in Section 3.2, treatment A will be assigned to subject $(n+1)$ with covariates z_{n+1} with probability

$$\varphi(\mathfrak{G}_n, Z_{n+1} = z_{n+1}) = \pi^0(\hat{\gamma}_n, z_{n+1}), \qquad n \geq 2n_0. \tag{6.46}$$

Assuming that the target function π^0 is differentiable in γ under the expectation functional, with bounded derivatives, Zhang et al. (2007b) have provided all the asymptotics for such a design, as well as the associated asymptotic inference. Indeed, let $N_n(z) = \sum_{i=1}^n \mathbb{1}_{\{Z_i = z\}}$ be the number of subjects with covariate profile z after n steps and $\pi_n(z) = \sum_{i=1}^n \delta_i \mathbb{1}_{\{Z_i = z\}} / \sum_{i=1}^n \mathbb{1}_{\{Z_i = z\}}$ the corresponding percentage of assignments to A, the authors have derived a Strong Law of Large Numbers for the allocation proportions, both marginally and conditionally on a given covariate level (provided that $\Pr(Z = z) > 0$),

$$\lim_{n\to\infty} \pi_n = E_Z[\pi^0(\gamma, z)] \quad a.s. \qquad \text{and} \qquad \lim_{n\to\infty} \pi_n(z) = \pi^0(\gamma, z) \quad a.s. \tag{6.47}$$

deriving also the asymptotic normality of π_n and $\pi_n(z)$. Moreover, the estimator $\hat{\gamma}_n$ is strongly consistent and asymptotically normal.

As shown for the SML design, the CARA design (6.46) too may be inefficient due to its strong variability, since the allocation rule

- depends on the past history of the trial only through the estimation of the parameters;
- randomizes assignments through the current estimate of the target relative to the current covariate profile, without making use of further information.

6.4.2 Covariate-adjusted Doubly-adaptive Biased Coin Design

In order to overcome the drawbacks of the Covariate-adjusted SML designs, Zhang and Hu (2009) have introduced a different class of CARA designs, called the Covariate-adjusted Doubly-adaptive Biased Coin Designs (CD-BCD), which force the assignments towards the target similarly to Eisele's D-BCD (see Section 3.4) and guarantee a smaller variability of the allocation proportion.

This procedure, which seems to be particularly useful in the context of continuous covariates, is defined by

$$\varphi(\mathfrak{G}_n, Z_{n+1} = z_{n+1}) = \frac{\pi^0(\hat{\gamma}_n, z_{n+1})\left(\frac{\hat{\rho}_n}{\pi_n}\right)^{\alpha}}{\pi^0(\hat{\gamma}_n, z_{n+1})\left(\frac{\hat{\rho}_n}{\pi_n}\right)^{\alpha} + (1 - \pi^0(\hat{\gamma}_n, z_{n+1}))\left(\frac{1-\hat{\rho}_n}{1-\pi_n}\right)^{\alpha}}, \tag{6.48}$$

where $\hat{\rho}_n = n^{-1}\sum_{i=1}^{n}\pi^0(\hat{\gamma}_n, \boldsymbol{z}_i)$ and the non-negative parameter α controls the degree of randomness of each allocation: if $\alpha \to 0$ the randomization function does not depend on the current allocation proportion and this design corresponds to (6.46), whereas as α grows the allocations tend to be deterministic.

The rationale behind this choice is the following: when the global allocation proportion π_n is close to $\hat{\rho}_n$, which is a consistent estimate of its corresponding asymptotic target $E_{\boldsymbol{Z}}[\pi^0(\boldsymbol{\gamma}, \boldsymbol{z})]$, then the assignment depends essentially on the current estimate of the target for the current subject's covariates; otherwise, the allocation is forced towards A increasingly as $\hat{\rho}_n/\pi_n$ grows, i.e. if A is under-represented with respect to its estimated target value.

Strong consistency and asymptotic normality of the estimators are guaranteed; moreover Zhang and Hu (2009) have provided the almost sure convergence as well as the asymptotic normality of π_n, also deriving the asymptotic variance of the design, which is a decreasing function of the randomization parameter α.

6.4.3 The Reinforced Doubly-adaptive Biased Coin Design

As shown previously, when the target allocation is a continuous function of the unknown parameters of the model, CARA procedures (6.46) and (6.48) may be adopted in order to gradually approach the desired target. However, in the context of categorical covariates the evolution as well as the convergence of the allocation proportion at each stratum depends on the number of subjects falling into that covariate profile, which is (on average) related to the representativeness of the stratum in the population of interest. So, covariate profiles that could potentially be under-represented might induce high deviation from the corresponding targets, and for small samples this could be critical, both from inferential and an ethical viewpoints.

For this reason, Baldi Antognini and Zagoraiou (2012) have proposed the Reinforced Doubly-adaptive Biased Coin Design (RD-BCD), which is a general class of CARA procedures for categorical covariates aimed at converging to any given allocation proportion by forcing closeness to the target when necessary.

Assume for simplicity that only two categorical covariates are of interest, $\boldsymbol{Z} = (T, W)$, and let $\boldsymbol{\pi}_n = [\pi_n(j,l); j = 0,\ldots,J; l = 0,\ldots,L]$ and $\boldsymbol{N}_n = [N_n(j,l); j = 0,\ldots,J; l = 0,\ldots,L]$. Let $\boldsymbol{\pi}^0 = [\pi^0(j,l) : j = 0,\ldots,J; l = 0,\ldots,L]$ be a desired allocation proportion such that at each stratum (j,l) the corresponding target $\pi^0(j,l) = \pi^0(j,l;\boldsymbol{\gamma},\boldsymbol{p}) \in (0,1)$ is a continuous function of the unknown parameters. The RD-BCD is defined as follows: after an initial stage with n_0 observations made on each treatment in order to obtain a non-trivial parameter estimation $\widehat{\boldsymbol{\gamma}}_{2n_0}$ and $\widehat{\boldsymbol{p}}_{2n_0}$, at each step $n > 2n_0$ let $\widehat{\boldsymbol{\pi}}_n^0 = \boldsymbol{\pi}^0(\widehat{\boldsymbol{\gamma}}_n, \widehat{\boldsymbol{p}}_n)$ be the estimate of the target obtained by all the data up to that step. The $(n+1)$th subject with covariate profile $\boldsymbol{Z}_{n+1} = (j,l)$ will be assigned to A with probability

$$\varphi\left(\pi_n(j,l); \widehat{\pi}_n^0(j,l); \hat{p}_{njl}\right), \tag{6.49}$$

where the function $\varphi(x,y,z) : (0,1)^3 \to [0,1]$ satisfies the following properties:

i) $\varphi(x,y,z)$ is decreasing in x and increasing in y, for all $z \in (0,1)$;

ii) $\varphi(x, x, z) = x$ for all $z \in (0, 1)$;

iii) $\varphi(x, y, z)$ is decreasing in z if $x < y$, and increasing in z if $x > y$;

iv) $\varphi(x, y, z) = 1 - \varphi(1 - x, 1 - y, z)$ for all $z \in (0, 1)$.

From conditions i) and ii), at each stratum the allocation proportion will be forced to the corresponding target, since $\varphi(x, y, z) \leq y$ when $x \geq y$ and $\varphi(x, y, z) \geq y$ if $x < y$ for all $z \in (0, 1)$. Furthermore, condition iii) means that the allocation is forced towards optimality increasingly as the representativeness of the strata decreases and iv) guarantees that the two treatments are treated symmetrically.

Remark 6.2 *The RD-BCD in (6.49) is a vast class of designs that admits also discontinuous randomization functions; so, it generalizes some of the existing procedures, for instance rule (6.46) and Atkinson's D_A-BCD (6.33); moreover, the RD-BCD extends Eisele's D-BCD (see Section 3.4) and the ERADE (see Section 3.5) to the case of covariates.*

The randomization function could also be chosen in a different way at each of the strata for discriminating their relative importance. For any such choice, the allocation proportions of the Reinforced Doubly-adaptive Biased Coin Design converge almost surely to the desired target, i.e.,

$$\lim_{n \to \infty} \boldsymbol{\pi}_n = \boldsymbol{\pi}^0 \qquad a.s. \tag{6.50}$$

Moreover, strong consistency and asymptotic normality of the estimators are ensured (see, for details, Baldi Antognini and Zagoraiou (2012)).

Baldi Antognini and Zagoraiou (2012) have suggested the following family of allocation functions:

$$\varphi(x; y; z) = \frac{F\left[D\left(x; y\right)^{H(z)} F^{-1}(y)\right]}{F\left[D(x; y)^{H(z)} F^{-1}(y)\right] + F\left[D(1 - x; 1 - y)^{H(z)} F^{-1}(1 - y)\right]}, \tag{6.51}$$

where

- $F : \mathbb{R}^+ \to \mathbb{R}^+$ is continuous and strictly increasing;
- $H(z)$ is a decreasing function that governs the amount of randomness in the different strata;
- $D(x; y) : (0; 1)^2 \to \mathbb{R}^+$ represents a dissimilarity measure between the actual allocation proportion x and the current estimate of the optimal target y, which is assumed to be decreasing in x and increasing in y, with $D(x; x) = 1$ for all $x \in (0, 1)$.

Example 6.4 *A special case is $D(x; y) = 1$ for all $(x, y) \in (0, 1)^2$, then (6.51) becomes*

$$\varphi(x; y; z) = y, \qquad \forall (x, z) \in (0, 1)^2, \tag{6.52}$$

which corresponds to the Covariate-adjusted SML design in (6.46).

Example 6.5 *Another special case is* $F(t) = t$, $D(x;y) = y/x$ *and* $H(z) = \alpha \geq 0$ $\forall z \in (0,1)$, *i.e.,*

$$\varphi(x;y;z) = \frac{y(y/x)^{\alpha}}{y(y/x)^{\alpha} + (1-y)[(1-y)/(1-x)]^{\alpha}}, \quad \forall z \in (0,1),$$

which gives a natural extension in the presence of covariates of the family of Doubly-adaptive BCD's, which differs from the Covariate-adjusted Doubly-adaptive Biased Coin Design in (6.48), since at each step the CD-BCD considers a dissimilarity measure between the actual allocation proportion $\pi_n(j,l)$ *and* $\hat{\rho}_n$, *instead of the current estimate of the target* $\widehat{\pi}_n^*(j,l)$ *itself.*

Example 6.6 *An example of discontinuous allocation function is obtained by letting* $F(t) = t$, $H(z) = \{(J+1)(L+1)z\}^{-1}$ *and*

$$D(x;y) = \begin{cases} 1+\varepsilon, & x < y \\ 1, & x = y, \\ 1-\varepsilon, & x > y \end{cases} \qquad \text{with} \quad \varepsilon \in [0,1) \quad ,$$

then (6.51) becomes

$$\varphi(x;y;z) = \begin{cases} \frac{y(1+\varepsilon)^{\{(J+1)(L+1)z\}^{-1}}}{y(1+\varepsilon)^{\{(J+1)(L+1)z\}^{-1}} + (1-y)(1-\varepsilon)^{\{(J+1)(L+1)z\}^{-1}}}, & x < y \\ y, & x = y \\ \frac{y(1-\varepsilon)^{\{(J+1)(L+1)z\}^{-1}}}{y(1-\varepsilon)^{\{(J+1)(L+1)z\}^{-1}} + (1-y)(1+\varepsilon)^{\{(J+1)(L+1)z\}^{-1}}}, & x > y \end{cases}, \tag{6.53}$$

which allows us to force the allocations towards the chosen target increasingly the more we move away from the uniform distribution of the covariates.

Example 6.7 *Another special case is when the optimal target is the jointly balanced allocation*

$$\boldsymbol{\pi}_I^* = [\pi_I^*(j,l) = 1/2, \ \textit{for all}\ j = 0,\ldots,J; l = 0,\ldots,L]. \tag{6.54}$$

Letting $F(t) = t^2$, $H(z) = 1$ *and* $D(x;y) = 1 - 2(x-y)$, *then (6.51) with* $y = 1/2$

$$\varphi(x;1/2;z) = \frac{(1-x)^2}{(1-x)^2 + x^2}$$

corresponds to Atkinson's D_A*-BCD (6.33), whereas procedure (6.53) becomes a stratified version of Efron's BCD, namely a special case of the C-ABCD in (6.34).*

We end this section by pointing out some research on CARA procedures that are covariate-balanced and tend to skew the allocation probabilities to the treatment that appears to be superior at each step; see Ning and Huang (2010) and Yuan et al. (2011). However, the importance of balancing the treatments across covariates when binary or logistic response models are assumed is not clear. Formal mathematical justifications for the asymptotic allocations generated by such procedures, and in general their asymptotic properties, are not available at the moment.

6.5 Combined optimal designs with covariates

In Chapter 5 we have investigated strategies for finding target allocations of the treatments that combine inferential demands and ethical concerns. In the present section we wish to extend the combined optimization approach involving efficiencies discussed in Section 5.5.2 to include the presence of categorical covariates and deal with a method for deriving optimal combined targets that depend on the covariates.

6.5.1 Ethical and inferential criteria

As shown in Section 6.2, from an ethical perspective it is crucial to consider statistical models that account for possible treatment/covariate interactions, like (6.12). Otherwise, in the simplified scenario of parallel treatment effects, the relative performances of the two treatments are constant for each covariate profile, so that the ethical goal consists simply in assigning the majority of subjects to the better treatment and the presence or absence of covariates becomes irrelevant (see Bandyopadhyay and Biswas (2001), Atkinson and Biswas (2005a), Atkinson and Biswas (2005b) and Bandyopadhyay et al. (2007)).

From an ethical viewpoint, the optimal design consists in allocating each patient to the better treatment. Clearly, assuming (6.12) the better treatment may change on the basis of the subject's characteristics and furthermore the effects of non-optimal allocations may be different over the strata. Assume for simplicity that only two categorical covariates are of interest, i.e., $\boldsymbol{Z} = (T, W)$. Since at each stratum the superiority or inferiority of a given treatment depends only on the sign of ς in (6.14), the ith subject with covariate profile $\boldsymbol{Z}_i = (j, l)$ is assigned to the best treatment if and only if

$$\delta_i \mathbb{1}_{\{\varsigma(j,l)>0\}} + (1-\delta_i)\mathbb{1}_{\{\varsigma(j,l)<0\}}$$

(when $\varsigma(j, l) = 0$ the two arms collapse and every allocation is equivalent) and thus the proportion of subjects within this stratum receiving the best treatment is

$$\breve{\mathcal{E}}\left(\pi(j,l)\right) = \begin{cases} \pi(j,l) & \text{if } \varsigma(j,l) > 0, \\ 1-\pi(j,l) & \text{if } \varsigma(j,l) < 0, \end{cases} \tag{6.55}$$

(see the analogy with the ethical loss measured by criterion $\mathcal{E}$ in (5.3)). Thus, a reasonable (global) ethical measure suggested by Baldi Antognini and Zagoraiou (2012) is

$$\breve{\mathcal{E}}(\boldsymbol{\pi}_n, \boldsymbol{N}_n) = \frac{1}{n}\sum_{j=0}^{J}\sum_{l=0}^{L} N_n(j,l)|\varsigma(j,l)|\breve{\mathcal{E}}\left(\pi(j,l)\right), \tag{6.56}$$

which can be regarded as the percentage of correct choices suitably weighed by the relative ethical gain. Obviously, the ethically optimal target that assigns all the subjects to the better treatment is

$$\pi^*_{\mathcal{E}} = \left[\pi^*_{\mathcal{E}}(j,l) = \frac{1+\operatorname{sgn}(\varsigma(j,l))}{2};\ \text{for all } j = 0,\dots,J; l = 0,\dots,L\right], \tag{6.57}$$

which depends on the unknown model parameters.

Remark 6.3 *Without treatment/covariate interactions, at each stratum (j,l) we have $\zeta(j,l) = \mu_A - \mu_B$, so that criterion (6.56) becomes*

$$\breve{\mathcal{E}}(\boldsymbol{\pi}_n, \boldsymbol{N}_n) = (\mu_A - \mu_B)\left(\mathbb{1}_{\{\mu_A - \mu_B > 0\}} - 1 + \pi_n\right),$$

that depends on the design only through the global proportion π_n of assignments to A. Thus, under (6.1) the covariates are irrelevant from the utility viewpoint.

Taking into account inference, the fundamental measures of efficiency are the optimality criteria (6.22) through (6.25) of Section 6.2.3. They depend on the design only through $\boldsymbol{\pi}_n$ and also depend on the random covariates through the number of subjects within the different strata $\boldsymbol{N}_n$, that is, $\Phi(\boldsymbol{\pi}_n, \boldsymbol{N}_n)$. Moreover, criteria (6.22) through (6.25) are strictly convex in $\boldsymbol{\pi}_n$ and are minimized by the jointly balanced design

$$\boldsymbol{\pi}_{\mathcal{I}}^* = [\pi_{\mathcal{I}}^*(j,l) = 1/2, \text{ for all } j = 0, \dots, J; l = 0, \dots, L], \tag{6.58}$$

independently of the covariates.

Due to the dependence on $\boldsymbol{N}_n$, ethical criterion (6.56) and inferential criteria (6.22) through (6.25) are random quantities; to obtain suitable design measures by removing the random effect induced by the covariates, a possible solution consists in taking their expected values, namely

$$\ddot{\mathcal{E}}(\boldsymbol{\pi}_n) = E_{\boldsymbol{Z}}[\breve{\mathcal{E}}(\boldsymbol{\pi}_n, \boldsymbol{N}_n)] \quad \text{and} \quad \ddot{\Phi}(\boldsymbol{\pi}_n) = E_{\boldsymbol{Z}}[\Phi(\boldsymbol{\pi}_n, \boldsymbol{N}_n)]. \tag{6.59}$$

6.5.2 Compound optimal allocations

As in Chapter 5, consider a compromise criterion of the following form:

$$\Psi_\omega(\boldsymbol{\pi}_n) = \omega\left\{\frac{1}{\Psi_2(\boldsymbol{\pi}_n)}\right\} + (1-\omega)\left\{\frac{1}{\Psi_1(\boldsymbol{\pi}_n)}\right\}, \tag{6.60}$$

where ω is a weight that expresses an overall measure of risk for the population of interest, and

$$\Psi_2(\boldsymbol{\pi}_n) = \frac{\ddot{\mathcal{E}}(\boldsymbol{\pi}_n)}{\ddot{\mathcal{E}}(\boldsymbol{\pi}_{\mathcal{E}}^*)} \quad \text{and} \quad \Psi_1(\boldsymbol{\pi}_n) = \frac{\ddot{\Phi}(\boldsymbol{\pi}_{\mathcal{I}}^*)}{\ddot{\Phi}(\boldsymbol{\pi}_n)}. \tag{6.61}$$

are the standardized criteria of ethical and inferential efficiency that should be maximized.

The ethical weight ω can be set a priori by the experimenter but, in general, it is reasonable to define

$$\omega = \omega\left(E_{\boldsymbol{Z}}[|\zeta(\boldsymbol{z})|]\right) : \mathbb{R}^+ \cup \{0\} \to [0;1),$$

where ω is a a continuous and increasing function with $\omega(0) = 0$. Clearly the choice of the weight function depends on the given applied context and the available information. For instance, when the ethical costs are moderate more attention should be dedicated to inference, so that ω can be chosen to be an S-shaped function; whereas, in the case of possible serious adverse events ω can be modelled so as to increase very rapidly. Baldi Antognini and Zagoraiou (2012) have obtained the following result:

Theorem 6.3 *For every inferential criterion (6.22)-(6.25), there exists a unique target allocation* $\boldsymbol{\pi}^*_\omega = [\pi^*_\omega(j,l); j = 0,\ldots,J; l = 0,\ldots,L]$ *minimizing criterion* Ψ_ω *in (6.60), which is the solution of the following set of equations*

$$\left[\ddot{\mathcal{E}}(\boldsymbol{\pi}_n)\right]^2 \frac{\partial\ddot{\Phi}(\boldsymbol{\pi}_n)}{\partial\pi_n(j,l)} = \left(\frac{\omega}{1-\omega}\right)\ddot{\mathcal{E}}(\boldsymbol{\pi}^*_{\mathcal{E}})\ddot{\Phi}(\boldsymbol{\pi}^*_{\mathcal{I}})\zeta(j,l)p_{jl}, \qquad \forall(j,l). \tag{6.62}$$

At each stratum (j,l)*, the optimal combined target* $\pi^*_\omega(j,l)$ *satisfies the following properties:*

i) $\pi^*_\omega(j,l) = \pi^*_\omega(j,l;\gamma,\mathbf{p})$ *is a continuous function of* γ *and* $\mathbf{p}$*, with* $\pi^*_\omega(j,l;\gamma,\mathbf{p}) \in (0;1)$*;*

ii) $\pi^*_\omega(j,l;\gamma,\mathbf{p})$ *is increasing in* $\zeta(j,l)$ *for any given covariate distribution* $\mathbf{p}$*;*

iii) if γ' *and* γ'' *are two different set of parameter values with corresponding ethical gains* $\zeta'(j,l) = -\zeta''(j,l)$*, then for any given* $\mathbf{p}$

$$\pi^*_\omega(j,l;\gamma',\mathbf{p}) = 1 - \pi^*_\omega(j,l;\gamma'',\mathbf{p}); \tag{6.63}$$

iv) if $\zeta(j,l) > 0$ *(or* < 0*) then* $\pi^*_\omega(j,l;\gamma,\mathbf{p})$ *is increasing (respectively decreasing) in* p_{jl}*.*

Properties ii) and iii) mean that the optimal combined target is ethically feasible: first of all in each stratum it always assigns more than half the subjects to the better treatment and the allocation to the better treatment increases in the expected treatment difference. Property iv) means that the optimal combined target forces the allocation to the better treatment increasingly as the representativeness of the stratum increases, whereas property i) guarantees that suitable CARA procedures, like those discussed in Section 6.4, can be adopted in order to converge to $\pi^*_\omega(j,l)$.

6.6 Other adaptive designs with covariates

In this chapter we have only considered particular cases of the linear homoscedastic model, but different statistical models, which in general are special cases of the generalized linear model, are needed to describe other very common types of responses, for example, binary outcomes, survival outcomes and time-to-event data, when covariates are also observed. Suggestions of adaptive designs for such data can be found in the book by Atkinson and Biswas (2014), and here we mention a few. The theoretical results available at present are scarce.

6.6.1 Atkinson's Biased Coin Design for heteroscedastic normal models with covariates

Set the response variance under treatment j to be σ_j^2 $(j = A, B)$. Model (6.1) becomes

$$E[Y_i] = \delta_i \mu_A + (1-\delta_i)\mu_B + \boldsymbol{h}(\boldsymbol{z}_i)^t \boldsymbol{\beta}, \qquad Var[Y_i] = \delta_i \sigma_A^2 + (1-\delta_i)\sigma_B^2 \qquad i \geq 1.$$

With heteroscedastic observations, assuming the variances known, estimation is by Weighted Least Squares. If the variances are unknown, they are estimated sequentially. Atkinson and Biswas (2014) update the adaptive allocation rule of Atkinson's D_A-BCD with covariates replacing the allocation probability of treatment A in (6.31) by

$$\Pr(\delta_{n+1} = 1 \mid \Im_n, \boldsymbol{z}_{n+1}) = \frac{\tilde{d}(A, n, \boldsymbol{z}_{n+1})/\sigma_A}{\tilde{d}(A, n, \boldsymbol{z}_{n+1})/\sigma_A + \tilde{d}(B, n, \boldsymbol{z}_{n+1})/\sigma_B}, \tag{6.64}$$

where $\tilde{d}(j, n, \boldsymbol{z}_{n+1}) = \left(1 - (1; \boldsymbol{h}(\boldsymbol{z}_{n+1})^t)(\mathbb{F}_n^t \mathbb{F}_n)^{-1} \boldsymbol{b}_n\right)^2$.

There is also a Bayesian version, with (6.64) replaced by

$$\Pr(\delta_{n+1} = 1 \mid \Im_n, \boldsymbol{z}_{n+1}) = $$
$$= \frac{\sigma_A \left(1 + \tilde{d}(A, n, \boldsymbol{z}_{n+1})/\sigma_A^2\right)^{1/v}}{\sigma_A \left(1 + \tilde{d}(A, n, \boldsymbol{z}_{n+1})/\sigma_A^2\right)^{1/v} + \sigma_B \left(1 + \tilde{d}(B, n, \boldsymbol{z}_{n+1})/\sigma_B^2\right)^{1/v}}$$

where v has the same meaning as in Section 4.7. No further details are provided, but some numerical comparisons are performed.

6.6.2 Atkinson's Biased Coin Design for binary data with covariates

If the probabilities of success p_j $(j = A, B)$ under the different treatments depend on covariates as follows

$$\log\left(\frac{p_j}{1-p_j}\right) = \mu_j + \boldsymbol{h}(\boldsymbol{z})^t \boldsymbol{\beta},$$

the suggestion in Atkinson and Biswas (2014) is to assign the $(n+1)$th subject to treatment A with probabilities

$$\frac{\tilde{d}(A, n, \boldsymbol{z}_{n+1})/\sqrt{p_A(1-p_A)}}{\sum_{s=1}^{2} \tilde{d}(s, n, \boldsymbol{z}_{n+1})/\sqrt{p_s(1-p_s)}} \tag{6.65}$$

and this suggestion is again matched by the outcome of some simulations. However in (6.65), p_j depends on the unknown μ_A, μ_B and $\boldsymbol{\beta}$, which must be estimated sequentially, and on the observed covariate $\boldsymbol{z}_{n+1}$.

6.6.3 Randomized Play-the-Winner and Drop-the-Loser with covariates

Possible approaches to the introduction of covariates in urn designs have been given by Bandyopadhyay and Biswas (1997b) and Bandyopadhyay et al. (2009), and can be found in Atkinson and Biswas (2014). For binary responses and one covariate (prognostic factor) z with levels $u = 0, 1, \ldots, J$ ordered from the least to the most favourable condition, it is assumed that

$$\Pr(Y_i = 1) = [p_A \delta_i + p_B(1 - \delta_i)]\, a^{J-u}, \qquad i \geq 1, \tag{6.66}$$

where u is the covariate level of the ith subject and $a \in (0;1)$ is a *prognostic factor index*, assumed known. The treatment of an entering subject at grade u is determined by drawing a ball, which is then replaced into the urn together with another $(J-u+r)\beta$ balls of the same type and $u\beta$ of the opposite type if success is observed. In case of failure, we add $(J-u)\beta$ balls of the same kind and $(u+r)\beta$ of the opposite kind: r is a design parameter meant to give more weight to a success for a subject with a less favourable prognosis. Under appropriate hypotheses the authors calculate the limiting proportion of subjects receiving treatments A and B, which does not depend on β, but will depend on r.

Under the same assumption (6.66), Bandyopadhyay et al. (2009) provide the covariate-adjusted version of Drop-the-Loser. A set of probabilities are chosen a priori: $\pi_0 < \pi_1 < \ldots < \pi_J$. Then a treatment ball is replaced with probability π_j when a success has been observed at level j, whereas for a failure at the same level the ball is replaced with probability π_{J-j}. The handling of immigration balls is the same as for the DL. Again, the rationale is for responses with unfavourable prognostic factors to have a greater impact. The limit proportion of subjects receiving A is obtained.

In Bandyopadhyay and Bhattacharya (2012) the allocation procedures mentioned above are assessed both numerically and theoretically, and the performance of the design is also investigated in a related hypothetical clinical trial.

6.7 Some conclusions

It is clear from the previous sections that the theory of adaptive randomization with a full use of covariates has been debated in depth only for simple, i.e., normal homoscedastic, models. In particular, there is not yet a theory of compound optimal allocations for heteroscedastic outcomes. Due to its practical importance in applications, its extension appears to be a priority, also in the light of the modern advances in personalized medicine.

More in general, it is remarkable that the open problems highlighted in the conclusions of Hu and Rosenberger (2006) still appear to be the relevant ones, although some progress has been made in CARA randomization (see for instance Sections 6.3 through 6.5). Attention to urn models seems nowadays to be on the decline. On the other hand, adaptive designs for survival models have begun to be considered, while adaptive randomization for longitudinal data is still an open issue.

The list of topics that deserve a better understanding is long; we have hinted at some in the course of the book. For instance, theoretical work on the interplay between sequential analysis and adaptive randomization (in particular as regards finding a suitable stopping rule to match the chosen allocation rule) is scarce, possibly because of the mathematical complexity.

We hope that this book will encourage statistical research in all these areas.

Appendix A

Optimal designs

The classical theory of Optimal Designs deals with methods for choosing the best design for inference in the non-sequential case. Optimal Design theory was first developed by Jack Kiefer in the 1960s for parameter estimation under the linear model with second-order assumptions. Later, the theory has been extended to other models, mainly in the family of the generalized linear models. The planning of an experiment is seen as a decision problem (in the absence of data) which thus requires the specification of a loss function (an optimality criterion), reflecting the degree of failure of the experiment to achieve its aims in terms of precision of the estimates, power of the test, etc. The optimal experiment is the one whose design minimizes such loss. Although practical restrictions or considerations of robustness with respect to the model might prevent the researchers from implementing the optimum design, the choice of a criterion allows them to use the optimum as a benchmark against which to measure the efficiency of all the other designs.

To help the readability of the book, this appendix contains some basic definitions and results that are useful tools for the comprehension of the designs considered in our monograph. For a full understanding, we refer to the existing books on optimal designs, e.g., Fedorov (1972), Silvey (1980), Pukelsheim (2006), Atkinson et al. (2007) and Pronzato and Pazman (2013). We stress that the classical theory of Optimal Designs is for fixed sample size, non-sequential experiments.

Design criteria for linear models

In an experimental setting, often the variable under study Y is taken to depend on a vector $\boldsymbol{x}$ of regressors, indicating the levels of some experimental conditions set by the experimenter. The *linear model* is a set of assumptions on the outcome, denoted by $Y(\boldsymbol{x})$, namely

1. $E[Y(\boldsymbol{x})] = \mathbf{f}(\mathbf{x})^t\boldsymbol{\gamma} = \sum_{j=1}^{p} f_j(\boldsymbol{x})\gamma_j$, where $\boldsymbol{\gamma} = (\gamma_1, \dots, \gamma_p)^t$ are unknown parameters and $\mathbf{f}(\boldsymbol{x})^t = (f_1(\boldsymbol{x}), \dots, f_p(\boldsymbol{x}))$ is a known vector function.
2. $Var[Y(\boldsymbol{x})] = \sigma^2$, where the constant σ^2 is in general regarded as a nuisance.

3. Different observations are uncorrelated.

Each choice of $\boldsymbol{x}$ is referred to as a *design point*. The goal of the original theory of Optimal Design is to fix the levels of the experimental conditions, i.e., to choose a set of design points, and the proportion of observations to be taken at each of them, in order to estimate the unknown parameters of the model as precisely as possible.

If Y_i $(i = 1, \ldots, n)$ denotes the outcome of observation i at the design point $\boldsymbol{x}_i$ in an experiment with fixed sample size n, then the linear model assumptions yield (in matrix notation)

$$E[\mathbf{Y}] = \mathbf{X}\gamma \qquad Var[\mathbf{Y}] = \sigma^2 \mathbf{I}_n, \tag{A.1}$$

where $\mathbf{I}_n$ is the $n \times n$ identity matrix, $\mathbf{Y} = (Y_1, \ldots, Y_n)^t$, and $\mathbf{X} = (\mathbf{f}(\boldsymbol{x}_i)^t)$ is an $(n \times p)$-dimensional matrix, usually called *design matrix*. We write $\mathbf{X}_n$ when we wish to stress the number of observations.

A more detailed set of distributional assumptions results when the responses are assumed to be normal homoscedastic, namely

$$\mathbf{Y} \sim N(\mathbf{X}\gamma, \sigma^2 \mathbf{I}). \tag{A.2}$$

The vector parameters γ is usually estimated by Ordinary Least Squares (OLS), that under normality assumptions (A.2) coincide with maximum likelihood. If rank$(\mathbf{X}) = p$, the OLS estimates are

$$\hat{\gamma} = (\mathbf{X}^t\mathbf{X})^{-1}\mathbf{X}^t\mathbf{Y}$$

and the predicted response corresponding to an unobserved value of $\boldsymbol{x}$ is $\hat{Y}(\boldsymbol{x}) = \mathbf{f}(\boldsymbol{x})^t\hat{\gamma}$.

We often wish to choose an experimental design which makes the variance-covariance matrix $\mathbf{V} = Var\,[\hat{\gamma}]$ "smallest", where

$$\mathbf{V} = \sigma^2(\mathbf{X}^t\mathbf{X})^{-1} = \sigma^2 \left(\sum_{i=1}^{n} \mathbf{f}(\mathbf{x}_i)\mathbf{f}(\boldsymbol{x}_i)^t \right)^{-1}.$$

Should $\mathbf{X}^t\mathbf{X}$ be singular, it is in general possible to replace its inverse by the Moore–Penrose generalized inverse.

An optimality criterion is a measure of loss of information and is frequently chosen to be a function Ψ of the matrix $\mathbf{V}$. The optimal design is the one that minimizes criterion Ψ, which is usually a matrix convex increasing (with respect to Loewner's ordering) function of $\mathbf{V}$. Matrix

$$\mathbf{M} = n^{-1}\mathbf{X}^t\mathbf{X} = n^{-1}\sum_{i=1}^{n} \mathbf{f}(\mathbf{x}_i)\mathbf{f}(\boldsymbol{x}_i)^t$$

is the *normalized information matrix* of the design and corresponds, up to σ^{-2}, to the normalized Fisher information when the responses are normally distributed (see Chapter 1). It is a peculiarity of the linear model that this matrix does not depend on the parameters of interest. Clearly, since $\mathbf{V} = n^{-1}\sigma^2\mathbf{M}^{-1}$, we may also define an *information criterion* Φ by $\Phi(\mathbf{M}) = \Psi(\mathbf{V})$ and maximize Φ. By well-known matrix theory results, if Ψ is matrix convex and increasing in $\mathbf{V}$, then Φ is matrix convex decreasing in $\mathbf{M}$ and minimization of $\Psi(\mathbf{V})$ corresponds to maximization of $\Phi(\mathbf{M})$.

The best known and most widely used criteria of this type are:

i) A-**optimality**, also called the **trace criterion**, which minimizes the average variance of the OLS estimators $\hat{\gamma}$, namely

$$\operatorname{tr}\mathbf{V} = Var\,[\hat{\gamma}_1] + \ldots + Var\,[\hat{\gamma}_p] = \sigma^2 \operatorname{tr}(\mathbf{X}^t\mathbf{X})^{-1}.$$

Clearly here (and in what follows) σ^2 can be neglected.

ii) D-**optimality** is the best known and most widely used criterion, introduced by Wald (1943), aimed at minimizing

$$\det \mathbf{V} = \sigma^2 \det(\mathbf{X}^t\mathbf{X})^{-1} = \sigma^2 \left(\det(\mathbf{X}^t\mathbf{X})\right)^{-1}.$$

Clearly, that is equivalent to maximizing $\det \mathbf{M}$ or $\log\det \mathbf{M}$. Under normality assumptions, $(1-\alpha)$-confidence ellipsoids for γ have the form

$$(\gamma - \hat{\gamma})^t(\mathbf{X}^t\mathbf{X})^{-1}(\gamma - \hat{\gamma}) \leq k_\alpha,$$

with k_α a suitable constant, and since the volume is proportional to $(\mathbf{X}^t\mathbf{X})^{-1/2}$, D-optimality minimizes this volume. Moreover, D-optimality is also equivalent to maximizing the power of the F-test of equality of the parameters. D-optimality is invariant under linear reparametrizations, whereas the trace criterion is invariant only with respect to orthogonal transformations of the parameters. The quantity $\det\left(\mathbf{X}^t\mathbf{X}\right)^{-1}$ is called the *generalized variance*. A useful result for the sequential construction of D-optimal designs is

$$\det(\mathbf{X}_{n+1}^t\mathbf{X}_{n+1}) = \det\left(\mathbf{X}_n^t\mathbf{X}_n\right)[1 + \mathbf{f}(\mathbf{x}_{n+1})^t \left(\mathbf{X}_n^t\mathbf{X}_n\right)^{-1}\mathbf{f}(\boldsymbol{x}_{n+1})]. \quad \text{(A.3)}$$

iii) E-**optimality**: if we are interested in all the linear combinations of the parameters, we may want to minimize the largest variance of $\mathbf{c}^t\gamma$ over all $\mathbf{c} \in \mathbb{R}^p$ such that $\mathbf{c}^t\mathbf{c} = 1$. Now

$$\begin{aligned}
\max_{\mathbf{c}^t\mathbf{c}=1} Var[\mathbf{c}^t\gamma] &= \max_{\mathbf{c}^t\mathbf{c}=1} \left(\sigma^2\mathbf{c}^t(\mathbf{X}^t\mathbf{X})^{-1}\mathbf{c}\right) \\
&= \text{max eigenvalue of } \sigma^2(\mathbf{X}^t\mathbf{X})^{-1} \\
&= \sigma^2(\text{min eigenvalue of } \mathbf{X}^t\mathbf{X})^{-1}.
\end{aligned}$$

Thus this criterion consists in maximizing the minimum eigenvalue of $\mathbf{X}^t\mathbf{X}$.

iv) c-**optimality**: if we are interested in estimating one particular linear combination $\mathbf{c}^t\gamma$ of the parameters (typically a difference), we may want to minimize $Var\,[\mathbf{c}^t\hat{\gamma}]$, that (up to the scalar σ^2) equals

$$\mathbf{c}^t(\mathbf{X}^t\mathbf{X})^{-1}\mathbf{c}\,.$$

A special case is if we are interested in predicting Y at a particular design point $\boldsymbol{x}_0$ of the design region and want to choose a design so as to minimize the variance of the predicted response at $\boldsymbol{x}_0$, since $Var[\hat{Y}(\boldsymbol{x}_0)] = \sigma^2 \mathbf{f}(\boldsymbol{x}_0)^t(\mathbf{X}^t\mathbf{X})^{-1}\mathbf{f}(\boldsymbol{x}_0)$. The quantity

$$d(\boldsymbol{x}_0, n) = \mathbf{f}(\boldsymbol{x}_0)^t(\mathbf{X}^t\mathbf{X})^{-1}\mathbf{f}(\boldsymbol{x}_0)$$

is called the *generalized variance* of the predicted response.

v) **Linear optimality** (also L-**optimality**) is obtained by extending the c-optimality criterion so as to deal with more than one function of the parameters, say $\mathbf{L}^t\boldsymbol{\gamma}$. Since $Var\left[\mathbf{L}^t\gamma\right] = \sigma^2\mathbf{L}^t(\mathbf{X}^t\mathbf{X})^{-1}\mathbf{L}$, the criterion is minimizing the sum of the variances (up to the scalar σ^2), namely minimizing

$$\operatorname{tr}\left(\mathbf{L}^t(\mathbf{X}^t\mathbf{X})^{-1}\mathbf{L}\right) = \operatorname{tr}\left((\mathbf{X}^t\mathbf{X})^{-1}\mathbf{L}\mathbf{L}^t\right).$$

We obtain the same criterion if we are interested in predicting Y over an entire design region $\mathfrak{X}$ and want to choose a design so as to minimize the average variance of the predicted response. Indeed, since

$$Var[\hat{Y}(\boldsymbol{x})] = \sigma^2\mathbf{f}(\boldsymbol{x})^t(\mathbf{X}^t\mathbf{X})^{-1}\mathbf{f}(\boldsymbol{x}),$$

then we minimize

$$\int_{\mathfrak{X}} \mathbf{f}(\boldsymbol{x})^t(\mathbf{X}^t\mathbf{X})^{-1}\mathbf{f}(\boldsymbol{x})d\boldsymbol{x} = \operatorname{tr}\left((\mathbf{X}^t\mathbf{X})^{-1}\int_{\mathfrak{X}}\mathbf{f}(\boldsymbol{x})\mathbf{f}(\boldsymbol{x})^t d\boldsymbol{x}\right),$$

where $\int_{\mathfrak{X}}\mathbf{f}(\boldsymbol{x})\mathbf{f}(\boldsymbol{x})^t d\boldsymbol{x}$ is a non-negative definite matrix.

vi) Instead of the trace, we can consider the determinant; and the criterion may be called D_L-**optimality**. The generalized variance of the predicted response is now

$$d_L(\boldsymbol{x}_0, n) = \mathbf{f}(\boldsymbol{x}_0)^t(\mathbf{X}^t\mathbf{X})^{-1}\mathbf{L}\left(\mathbf{L}^t(\mathbf{X}^t\mathbf{X})^{-1}\mathbf{L}\right)^{-1}\mathbf{L}^t\left(\mathbf{X}^t\mathbf{X}\right)^{-1}\mathbf{f}(\boldsymbol{x}_0).$$

In the sequential construction of D_L-optimum designs, formula (A.3) is replaced by

$$\det\left(\mathbf{L}^t(\mathbf{X}^t_{n+1}\mathbf{X}_{n+1})^{-1}\mathbf{L}\right)^{-1} = \det\left(\mathbf{X}^t_n\mathbf{X}_n\right)\times$$
$$\left[1+\mathbf{f}(\mathbf{x}_{n+1})^t\left(\mathbf{X}^t_n\mathbf{X}_n\right)^{-1}\mathbf{L}\left(\mathbf{L}^t(\mathbf{X}^t_n\mathbf{X}_n)^{-1}\mathbf{L}\right)^{-1}\mathbf{L}^t\left(\mathbf{X}^t_n\mathbf{X}_n\right)^{-1}\mathbf{f}(\boldsymbol{x}_{n+1})\right].$$

vii) Supposing we are interested in estimating only s parameters, say $\boldsymbol{\theta} = \left(\mathbf{I}_s : \mathbf{0}_{s\times(p-s)}\right)\boldsymbol{\gamma}$, where $\mathbf{0}_{s\times(p-s)}$ is a matrix of all zeroes, then the variance-covariance matrix of $\hat{\boldsymbol{\theta}}$ is

$$Var\left[\hat{\boldsymbol{\theta}}\right] = \sigma^2\left(\mathbf{I}_s : \mathbf{0}_{s\times(p-s)}\right)^t\left(\mathbf{X}^t\mathbf{X}\right)^{-1}\left(\mathbf{I}_s : \mathbf{0}_{s\times(p-s)}\right),$$

so $(\mathbf{X}^t\mathbf{X})^{-1}$ must be replaced by $\left(\mathbf{I}_s : \mathbf{0}_{s\times(p-s)}\right)^t(\mathbf{X}^t\mathbf{X})^{-1}\left(\mathbf{I}_s : \mathbf{0}_{s\times(p-s)}\right)$. If we decompose the matrix $\mathbf{X}$ as $\mathbf{X} = (\mathbf{X}_1 \colon \mathbf{X}_2)$, where $\mathbf{X}_1$ is $n \times s$ -dimensional and $\mathbf{X}_2$ is $n \times (p - s)$, then

$$\left(\mathbf{I}_s : \mathbf{0}_{s\times(p-s)}\right)^t (\mathbf{X}^t\mathbf{X})^{-1} \left(\mathbf{I}_s : \mathbf{0}_{s\times(p-s)}\right)$$
$$= \left(\mathbf{X}_1^t\mathbf{X}_1 - \mathbf{X}_1^t\mathbf{X}_2\left(\mathbf{X}_2^t\mathbf{X}_2\right)^{-1}\mathbf{X}_2^t\mathbf{X}_1\right)^{-1} \tag{A.4}$$

and A_s-**optimality**, D_s-**optimality**, etc. are defined as the corresponding $A-, D-$ etc. optimality criteria applied to matrix (A.4) or to the information matrix $\mathbf{X}_1^t\mathbf{X}_1 - \mathbf{X}_1^t\mathbf{X}_2\left(\mathbf{X}_2^t\mathbf{X}_2\right)^{-1}\mathbf{X}_2^t\mathbf{X}_1$.

In point of fact, A_s-optimality and D_s-optimality are special cases of L- and D_L-optimality with $\mathbf{L} = \left(\mathbf{I}_s : \mathbf{0}_{s\times(p-s)}\right)$.

Example A.1 *In a comparative experiments with two treatments without covariates, the model may simply be*

$$E[Y_i] = \delta_i\mu_1 + (1-\delta_i)\mu_2, \qquad Var[Y_i] = \sigma^2, \qquad i \geq 1, \tag{A.5}$$

so the generalized variance of the predicted response corresponding to treatment $j = A, B$ *after* n *steps is*

$$d(j, n) = \frac{1}{n_j}.$$

This is relevant for the D_A*-BCD of Section 2.6 in Chapter 2. If the allocation probabilities of* A *and* B *are proportional to* n_A^{-1} *and* n_B^{-1} *respectively, they must be equal to* n_B/n *and* n_A/n *respectively.*

Example A.2 *For the same model as Example A.1 the treatment difference is obtained with* $\mathbf{c} = (1; -1)^t$. *For treatment* A, $\boldsymbol{x}_{n+1} = (1; 0)^t$ *and*

$$d_L(A, n) = \mathbf{f}(\mathbf{x}_{n+1})^t \left(\mathbf{X}_n^t\mathbf{X}_n\right)^{-1}\mathbf{c}\left(\mathbf{c}^t(\mathbf{X}_n^t\mathbf{X}_n)^{-1}\mathbf{c}\right)^{-1}\mathbf{c}^t\left(\mathbf{X}_n^t\mathbf{X}_n\right)^{-1}\mathbf{f}(\boldsymbol{x}_{n+1})$$
$$= \frac{n_B}{n \cdot n_A}.$$

Similarly $d_L(B, n) = n_A/(n \cdot n_B)$. *This is relevant for the* D_A*-BCD of Section 2.4.3 in Chapter 2. If the allocation probabilities of* A *and* B *are proportional to* n_B/n_A *and* n_A/n_B *respectively, they must be equal to*

$$\frac{n_B^2}{n_A^2 + n_B^2} \quad \text{and} \quad \frac{n_A^2}{n_A^2 + n_B^2},$$

respectively.

The following are further criteria of optimality, not considered in this book.

viii) G-**optimality**: if we are interested in predicting Y over the entire design region $\mathfrak{X}$ and want to choose a design so as to minimize the maximum variance of the prediction, the criterion to be minimized will be

$$\sup_{\boldsymbol{x}\in\mathfrak{X}} \mathbf{f}(\boldsymbol{x})^t(\mathbf{X}^t\mathbf{X})^{-1}\mathbf{f}(\boldsymbol{x}).$$

ix) MV-**optimality**. This is a minimax criterion, it minimizes the maximum variance of the estimates $\hat{\gamma}_j$, i.e., the largest entry on the main diagonal of $(\mathbf{X}^t\mathbf{X})^{-1}$.

x) T-**optimality** and KL-**optimality**. One of the criticisms usually made to the theory of Optimal Designs is that a particular model has to be assumed before designing the experiment, which in most cases means before having any data. Sometimes several competing models appear to be adequate for the same problem. In this case, a model has to be chosen after a discrimination hypothesis test and we may seek an optimal design for model selection. For normally distributed observations, an optimality design criterion for discriminating between two homoscedastic models is the T-criterion (Atkinson and Fedorov, 1975a,b), which maximizes the power of the F-test for lack of fit. When the rival models are nested and they differ by s parameters, another criterion for model discrimination is D_s-optimality. An extension to a more general distributional setup is the recently proposed *KL-criterion* based on the Kullback-Leibler divergence (Lopez-Fidalgo et al., 2007), which coincides with the T-optimality criterion when the observations are normally distributed.

Optimality of balance under a linear homoscedastic model

For comparative experiments a *balanced* design is often regarded as desirable, and indeed under a linear homoscedastic model balance is often optimal with respect to a wide class of criteria, although the term "balance" has different meanings for different specifications of the model. Jack Kiefer was the first to prove instances of this optimality using invariance of the information matrix with respect to suitable permutations of the parameters: any permutation of the parameters induces a permutation on the rows and (the same) on columns of the matrix $\mathbf{X}^t\mathbf{X}$. Roughly speaking, a design can be denoted as **balanced** when its normalized information matrix $\mathbf{M}$ is invariant under a suitable group $\mathcal{G}$ of permutations operating simultaneously on the rows and columns. According to the particular problem under examination, different groups of permutations must be called for. Furthermore, apart from permutations, other matrix transformations are of relevance when investigating design optimality for the linear model: an in-depth study of this topic can be found in Giovagnoli et al. (1987). The invariance of $\mathbf{M}$ (and hence of the variance-covariance matrix $\mathbf{V}$) with respect to $\mathcal{G}$ is clearly necessary for optimality with respect to all the criteria Φ or Ψ satisfying the conditions

a) Φ is matrix convex in $\mathbf{M}$ (Ψ is matrix convex in $\mathbf{V}$),

b) Φ (Ψ) is invariant under permutations in $\mathcal{G}$,

since for all $0 < a < 1$ and permutation matrix Π

$$\Phi\left(a\mathbf{X}^t\mathbf{X} + (1-a)\Pi^t\mathbf{X}^t\mathbf{X}\Pi\right) \le a\Phi\left(\mathbf{X}^t\mathbf{X}\right) + (1-a)\Phi\left(\Pi^t\mathbf{X}^t\mathbf{X}\Pi\right) = \Phi\left(\mathbf{X}^t\mathbf{X}\right).$$

All the above criteria from i) to ix) satisfy condition **a)**; as long as in ii) we take $\Phi = -\log\det$. Criteria i) through iii), and also ix), are invariant with respect to any permutations of all the parameters. Criterion v), of which iv) is a special case, is invariant with respect to permutations of the parameters (hence of the rows of $\mathbf{L}$), that leave the matrix $\mathbf{L}\mathbf{L}^t$ invariant. The criteria considered in vi) are left invariant by the corresponding permutations of the s parameters of interest among themselves which fix the $p-s$ remaining parameters.

However invariance of the design does not always guarantee optimality. Since all the criteria of interest also satisfy

c) Φ is decreasing in $\mathbf{M}$ (Ψ is increasing in $\mathbf{V}$) with respect to the Loewner ordering,

as well as invariant the matrix $\mathbf{M}$ must also be minimal with respect to such ordering in the class of design information matrices we are considering. But if the invariant matrix is unique in that class, then it is straightforward that it must be optimal.

We now give a few examples of interest for comparative experiments with v treatments.

Example A.3 *Treatment estimation: when the model is simply*

$$E[Y_i] = \delta_i^t \boldsymbol{\mu}, \qquad Var[Y_i] = \sigma^2, \qquad i \geq 1, \tag{A.6}$$

the normalized information matrix is

$$\mathbf{M} = n^{-1}\mathbf{X}^t\mathbf{X} = n^{-1}diag(n_1, n_2, \ldots, n_v).$$

For fixed n, the invariance condition is $n_1 = n_2 = \ldots = n_v$. Since tr $(\mathbf{M}) = 1$ is fixed, the invariant matrix is unique and thus the equireplicated design is optimal with respect to $A-$, $D-$, $E-$ and $MV-$optimality.

Example A.4 *Treatment estimation with nuisance parameters $\boldsymbol{\beta} = (\beta_1, \ldots, \beta_p)^t$: if the model is*

$$E[\mathbf{Y}] = \boldsymbol{\Delta}\boldsymbol{\mu} + \mathbf{X}_2\boldsymbol{\beta}, \qquad Var[\mathbf{Y}] = \sigma^2\mathbf{I}_n, \tag{A.7}$$

where $\boldsymbol{\Delta} = (\boldsymbol{\delta}_1; \ldots; \boldsymbol{\delta}_n)^t$ and interest is in estimating only $\boldsymbol{\mu}$, the information for $\boldsymbol{\mu}$ is

$$\mathbf{M} = n^{-1}\left[\boldsymbol{\Delta}^t\boldsymbol{\Delta} - \boldsymbol{\Delta}^t\mathbf{X}_2\left(\mathbf{X}_2^t\mathbf{X}_2\right)^{-1}\mathbf{X}_2^t\boldsymbol{\Delta}\right]. \tag{A.8}$$

The invariance of (A.8) with respect to all the permutations of treatment parameters is ensured by the following two conditions holding simultaneously

$$\boldsymbol{\Delta}^t\boldsymbol{\Delta} = \frac{n}{v}\mathbf{I}_v \tag{A.9}$$

$$\left(\boldsymbol{\Delta}^t - \frac{1}{n}\mathbf{J}_{v\times n}\right)\mathbf{X}_2 = \mathbf{0}_{v\times p} \tag{A.10}$$

where $\mathbf{J}_{v\times n} = \mathbf{1}_v\mathbf{1}_n^t$ is a matrix of all ones. For given $\mathbf{X}_2$ the invariant information matrix is

$$\frac{n}{v}\mathbf{I}_v - \frac{1}{n}\mathbf{J}_v\left(\mathbf{1}_v^t\mathbf{X}_2\left(\mathbf{X}_2^t\mathbf{X}_2\right)^{-1}\mathbf{X}_2^t\mathbf{1}_v\right)$$

and thus is unique, and this is sufficient to ensure A_s- and D_s- optimality of the balanced design.

Example A.5 *Estimating treatment contrasts: assume*

$$E[\mathbf{Y}] = \mathbf{\Delta}\boldsymbol{\mu}, \qquad Var[\mathbf{Y}] = \sigma^2 \mathbf{I}_n \tag{A.11}$$

and let the contrasts of interest be $\mathbf{L}^t\boldsymbol{\mu} = (\mu_1 - \mu_2, \mu_1 - \mu_3, \ldots, \mu_1 - \mu_v)^t$. *In this case L-optimality, i.e., minimizing*

$$\frac{v-1}{n_1} + \frac{1}{n_2} + \ldots + \frac{1}{n_v}$$

is invariant with respect to any permutation of the last $v-1$ *treatments that leaves the first treatment fixed, so these treatments must be equireplicated for balance. However, for optimality we need* $n_1 = \sqrt{(v-1)}n_2$. *In the case of just two treatments, namely for estimating the contrast* $\mu_1 - \mu_2$, *permuting the two treatments leaves L-optimality invariant, so it is enough that the two treatments be equireplicated.*

Example A.6 *The case of two treatments in the presence of covariates that do not interact with the treatments: this is a special case of Example A.4. Let the model be*

$$E[\mathbf{Y}] = \mathbf{X}\boldsymbol{\gamma} = \boldsymbol{\delta}^{(n)}\mu_A + (\mathbf{1}_n - \boldsymbol{\delta}^{(n)})\mu_B + \mathbf{F}_n\boldsymbol{\beta}, \quad Var[\mathbf{Y}] = \sigma^2\mathbf{I}_n, \tag{A.12}$$

where μ_A *and* μ_B *are the treatment effects,* $\boldsymbol{\beta}$ *is a p-dimensional vector of covariate effects which may include interactions among the covariates,* $\mathbf{F}_n = (\boldsymbol{h}(\mathbf{z}_i)^t)_{n\times p}$ *with* $\mathbf{z}_i$ *the vector of covariates observed on the ith unit and* $\boldsymbol{h}(\cdot)$ *a known vector function. Here* $\mathbf{X} = (\boldsymbol{\delta}^{(n)}; \mathbf{1}_n - \boldsymbol{\delta}^{(n)}; \mathbf{F}_n)$, $\boldsymbol{\gamma}^t = (\mu_A, \mu_B, \boldsymbol{\beta}^t)$ *and* $\mathbf{M}$, *i.e., the* $(2+p)$*-dim information matrix of the parameter vector* $\boldsymbol{\gamma}$, *given the covariates and the design is:*

$$\mathbf{M} = \frac{1}{n}\begin{pmatrix} \boldsymbol{\delta}^{(n)t}\boldsymbol{\delta}^{(n)} & \boldsymbol{\delta}^{(n)t}\left(\mathbf{1}_n - \boldsymbol{\delta}^{(n)}\right) & \boldsymbol{\delta}^{(n)t}\mathbf{F}_n \\ \left(\mathbf{1}_n - \boldsymbol{\delta}^{(n)}\right)^t\boldsymbol{\delta}^{(n)} & \left(\mathbf{1}_n - \boldsymbol{\delta}^{(n)}\right)^t\left(\mathbf{1}_n - \boldsymbol{\delta}^{(n)}\right) & \left(\mathbf{1}_n - \boldsymbol{\delta}^{(n)}\right)^t\mathbf{F}_n \\ \mathbf{F}_n^t\boldsymbol{\delta}^{(n)} & \mathbf{F}_n^t\left(\mathbf{1}_n - \boldsymbol{\delta}^{(n)}\right) & \mathbf{F}_n^t\mathbf{F}_n \end{pmatrix}$$

$$= \begin{pmatrix} \pi_n & 0 & n^{-1}\boldsymbol{\delta}^{(n)t}\mathbf{F}_n \\ 0 & 1-\pi_n & n^{-1}\left(\mathbf{1}_n - \boldsymbol{\delta}^{(n)}\right)^t\mathbf{F}_n \\ n^{-1}\mathbf{F}_n^t\boldsymbol{\delta}^{(n)} & n^{-1}\mathbf{F}_n^t\left(\mathbf{1}_n - \boldsymbol{\delta}^{(n)}\right) & n^{-1}\mathbf{F}_n^t\mathbf{F}_n \end{pmatrix}. \tag{A.13}$$

If the vector $\boldsymbol{\beta}$ *is considered to be a nuisance parameter and the inferential interest lies in estimating* (μ_A, μ_B) *or* $\mu_A - \mu_B$ *as precisely as possible, letting* $\mathbf{L}^t = (\mathbf{I}_2 : \mathbf{0}_{2\times p})$, *optimality criteria of interested are the following special cases of* A_s*- and* D_s*-optimality:*

$$tr\left(\mathbf{L}^t\mathbf{M}^{-1}\mathbf{L}\right), \tag{A.14}$$

or

$$\det\left(\mathbf{L}^t\mathbf{M}^{-1}\mathbf{L}\right), \tag{A.15}$$

with $\mathbf{M}^{-1}$ *replaced by the Moore–Penrose generalized inverse if needed.*

The balance conditions (A.9) and (A.10) become

$$\left(2\boldsymbol{\delta}^{(n)} - \mathbf{1}_n\right)^t(\mathbf{1}_n : \mathbf{F}_n) = \mathbf{0}_{1\times(p+1)}, \tag{A.16}$$

A design with this property is optimal for model (A.12) with respect to any convex criterion Φ of the information matrix $\mathbf{M}$ in (A.13) which is left invariant by the permutation of the treatments, namely of the first two rows and two columns simultaneously, like (A.14) and (A.15).

Example A.7 *Estimating the contrast between two treatments in the presence of covariates that may interact with the treatments. A model that accounts for treatment/covariate interactions is the homoscedastic one with*

$$E[Y_i] = \delta_i\mu_A + (1-\delta_i)\mu_B + \mathbf{h}(\mathbf{z}_i)^t\left(\delta_i\boldsymbol{\beta}_A + (1-\delta_i)\boldsymbol{\beta}_B\right), \qquad i \geq 1, \quad \text{(A.17)}$$

where $\boldsymbol{\beta}_A$ and $\boldsymbol{\beta}_B$ are d-dim vectors of possibly different regression parameters. The vector of unknown model parameters is now $\boldsymbol{\gamma} = (\mu_A, \mu_B, \boldsymbol{\beta}_A^t, \boldsymbol{\beta}_B^t)^t$ and the corresponding $(2+2d)$-dimensional information matrix is

$$\mathbf{M} = \begin{pmatrix} \pi_n & 0 & n^{-1}\delta^{(n)t}\mathbf{F}_n & \mathbf{0}_{1\times d} \\ 0 & 1-\pi_n & \mathbf{0}_{1\times d} & n^{-1}(\mathbf{1}_n - \delta^{(n)})^t\mathbf{F}_n \\ n^{-1}\mathbf{F}_n^t\delta^{(n)} & \mathbf{0}_{d\times 1} & n^{-1}\mathbf{F}_n^t\tilde{\boldsymbol{\Delta}}\mathbf{F}_n & \mathbf{0}_{d\times d} \\ \mathbf{0}_{d\times 1} & n^{-1}\mathbf{F}_n^t(\mathbf{1}_n - \delta^{(n)}) & \mathbf{0}_{d\times d} & n^{-1}\mathbf{F}_n^t(\mathbf{I}_n - \tilde{\boldsymbol{\Delta}})\mathbf{F}_n \end{pmatrix}, \quad \text{(A.18)}$$

where $\tilde{\boldsymbol{\Delta}} = diag\left(\delta^{(n)}\right)$. For model (A.17) the following balance conditions

$$\left(2\delta^{(n)} - \mathbf{1}_n\right)^t(\mathbf{1}_n : \mathbf{F}_n) = \mathbf{0}_{1\times(d+1)} \quad \text{(A.19)}$$

$$\mathbf{F}_n^t(2\tilde{\boldsymbol{\Delta}} - \mathbf{I}_n)\mathbf{F}_n = \mathbf{0}_{d\times d}. \quad \text{(A.20)}$$

ensure invariance with respect to permutations of the bottom two block rows and the two right-hand block columns, as well as the first two rows and columns. Given the covariates, hence given $\mathbf{F}_n$, the invariant matrix is unique, namely

$$\mathbf{M} = \begin{pmatrix} 1/2 & 0 & (2n)^{-1}\mathbf{1}_n^t\mathbf{F}_n & \mathbf{0}_{1\times d} \\ 0 & 1/2 & \mathbf{0}_{1\times d} & (2n)^{-1}\mathbf{1}_n^t\mathbf{F}_n \\ (2n)^{-1}\mathbf{F}_n^t & \mathbf{1}_n\mathbf{0}_{d\times 1} & n^{-1}\mathbf{F}_n^t\mathbf{F}_n & \mathbf{0}_{d\times d} \\ \mathbf{0}_{d\times 1} & (2n)^{-1}\mathbf{F}_n^t\mathbf{1}_n & \mathbf{0}_{d\times d} & n^{-1}\mathbf{F}_n^t\mathbf{F}_n \end{pmatrix};$$

thus a balanced design is optimal for model (A.17) with respect to any convex criterion Φ of the information matrix $\mathbf{M}$ in (A.18) left invariant by an exchange of the two treatments. Letting $\mathbf{D}^t = (\mathbf{0}_{2d\times 2} : \mathbf{I}_{2d})$, some inferential criteria of interest with these properties are

$$\det Var[\hat{\gamma}_n] = \frac{\sigma^2}{n}\det\left(\mathbf{M}^{-1}\right), \quad \text{(A.21)}$$

$$tr\,Var\left[\hat{\gamma}_n\right] = \frac{\sigma^2}{n}tr\left(\mathbf{M}^{-1}\right), \quad \text{(A.22)}$$

$$\det Var\left[\boldsymbol{\beta}_A^t, \boldsymbol{\beta}_B^t\right] = \frac{\sigma^2}{n}\det\left(\mathbf{D}^t\mathbf{M}^{-1}\mathbf{D}\right), \quad \text{(A.23)}$$

and

$$tr\,Var\left[\hat{\boldsymbol{\beta}}_A - \hat{\boldsymbol{\beta}}_B\right] = \frac{\sigma^2}{n}tr\left(\mathbf{D}^t\mathbf{M}^{-1}\mathbf{D}\right). \quad \text{(A.24)}$$

Optimal designs for non-linear models

Often the assumptions (A.1) underlying the linear model are violated, either because $E[Y(\boldsymbol{x})]$ is a non-linear function of the unknown parameters, or because $Var[Y(\boldsymbol{x})]$ is not constant, or because observations are not uncorrelated, or in other ways. A comprehensive book on designs for non-linear models is by Pronzato and Pazman (2013), which includes also some optimal designs.

Roughly, the same classic design criteria seen above are defined to be functions of the asymptotic variance-covariance matrix of suitable estimators of the parameters. It is assumed that, at least asymptotically, this variance-covariance matrix could be approximated by the inverse of Fisher's information matrix. Letting $\mathbf{M}$ be the normalized Fisher information, the optimal design will be such as to minimize a convex decreasing function $\Phi(\mathbf{M})$.

For non-linear models both matrices $\mathbf{M}$ and $\mathbf{V}$ will generally depend on some of the unknown parameters and minimization of the criterion gives rise to designs that are also functions of the parameters. They are called *locally optimal* and in order to be implemented, they need a guess value for the unknown parameters. An alternative approach is to proceed sequentially: at each step the information obtained from the accumulated data is used to estimate the parameters of the model and thus estimate the would-be optimal design. This estimate will direct the choice of the next design points and the procedure is then reiterated. This idea goes back to Silvey (1980); however, the actual optimality of this method with respect to the inferential criterion that has been chosen is not evident.

Lastly, the Bayesian paradigm can also be applied (see Appendix B).

Appendix B

Bayesian approaches in adaptive designs

As is well known, the Bayesian paradigm (Bernardo and Smith, 1994; Carlin and Louis, 2009) makes explicit use of *prior information* in the statistical analysis by treating the unknown parameters of the model as random quantities and expressing the a priori uncertainty about them by means of a probability distribution, the *prior*, which after observing the responses is updated to a *posterior* distribution via Bayes' theorem. The posterior is used to make inferences about the unknown quantities, and to calculate the *predictive* distribution of future observations given the past ones. The process may be iterated using the posterior distribution as the new prior. Randomization is not essential in Bayesian statistics, but it still plays a role, since biases that creep in may make legitimate conclusions impossible. In clinical trials in particular, Bayesians share with non-Bayesians the goal of randomizing patients to treatment arms so as to assign more patients to the treatments that do better in the trial.

The whole of Bayesian inference is conditional on the data: in other words, what matters are the actual observations, and the way in which the data were obtained is irrelevant. For example, the reason for stopping a trial affects frequentist but not Bayesian inference. So, a major difference from the frequentist approach is that in the Bayesian setup experiments can be altered in mid-course without affecting the analysis. This seems to justify a practice used to be common, namely an experimental design inspired by a frequentist rule followed by a Bayesian analysis of the data.

However, Barnard (1959) suggested that prior information can and should be incorporated into the design problem and his viewpoint has been taken up by a large number of authors and has percolated into practice. A much quoted overview of Bayesian design literature up to 1995 is Chaloner and Verdinelli (1995), but no update is yet available. Spiegelhalter et al. (2004), who devote Chapter 6 of their book to randomized controlled trials in a Bayesian perspective, deal explicitly with design and monitoring. The potential and adaptability of the Bayesian methodology in planning and conducting clinical researches is fully illustrated by Berry (2004), and indeed adaptive randomization in a Bayesian perspective has become a standard at some medical institutions, although the use of the Bayesian approach in the pharmaceutical developments is not widely accepted by the regulatory agencies. For non-sequential experiments, there are Bayesian design methods which have become classic by now: we describe them in the next section. A more thorough presentation is to be found in Piccinato (2009). More recently, hybrid approaches to experiments have been proposed which mix frequentist and Bayesian philosophies: inference is 100% frequentist, but a prior probability on the parameters is used to help the design stage. The rationale is that while a large number of statisticians would object to

Bayesian analysis on the grounds of its subjective nature, the same scientists would possibly agree on using prior information for choosing the experiment, since the choice takes place in the absence of data. This viewpoint may be thought of as a special case of the *design prior* versus *analysis prior* distinction that goes back to Etzioni and Kadane (1993): frequentist inference can often be obtained with a vague analysis prior.

It is true to say that sequential experimentation is, in general, congenial to the Bayesian methodology, and the present day interest in adaptive procedures has broadened the scope for theoretical developments of Bayesian designs too. In adaptive design theory, the idea of hybrid designs has become very popular: we have come across some of them in the rest of this book. No general theory of Bayesian adaptive designs exists yet, but Bayesian adaptive methods in clinical trials are the subject of the book by Berry et al. (2011), where Bayesian tools useful in early (Phase I), middle (Phase II) and late (Phase III) stage trials are presented. One section of that book (Section 4.4) is devoted to response-adaptive randomization. Some well-known adaptive Phase II studies, like BATTLE and the I-SPY TRIAL (see Berry et al. (2011)), were designed with a Bayesian approach.

The classic Bayesian theory in experimental designs

In the Bayesian setup, inference problems are often formulated in a decision theory framework. Let $\mathbf{y} = (y_1, \ldots, y_n)^t$ be the vector of responses and $\gamma \in \Omega$ the vector of unknown parameters of the model, with prior distribution $p(\gamma)$; let $d = d(\mathbf{y})$ denote a decision depending on the observed data (typically the estimate of a parameter, the choice between alternative hypotheses, or the choice between models), and let $W(d, \gamma)$ be a function that measures the loss of choosing d for each "true" value of the vector parameter γ. The *Bayes rule* is to take the decision that minimizes the *posterior risk*, i.e., the expected loss with respect to the posterior distribution $p(\gamma \mid \mathbf{y})$, namely

$$E_{\gamma|\mathbf{y}}[W(d(\mathbf{y}), \gamma) \mid \mathbf{y}]. \tag{B.1}$$

This concerns inference, but what about the experimental design? Lindley (1972) was the first to look at the choice of an experimental plan too as a statistical decision problem and defined an optimal Bayesian design to be the one which minimizes the *Bayes risk*, i.e., the loss incurred by the Bayes rule. Since at the design stage no data have been collected yet, evaluation of the design requires taking the expectation of (B.1) with respect to the marginal distribution of the responses

$$E_{\mathbf{Y}}[E_{\gamma|\mathbf{Y}}[W(d(\mathbf{Y}), \gamma)]].$$

Clearly the loss function can be replaced by a utility function and minimization by maximization.

When the purpose is to estimate γ under the assumption of a quadratic loss W, after the data $\mathbf{y} = (y_1, \ldots, y_n)^t$ have been observed the Bayes estimate is the posterior expectation $E[\gamma \mid \mathbf{y}]$ of γ, and the corresponding loss is the trace of the posterior covariance matrix, i.e., tr $Var[\gamma \mid \mathbf{y}]$: one needs to minimize the expected posterior loss $E[\mathrm{tr}\,Var[\gamma \mid \mathbf{y}]] = \mathrm{tr}\,E[Var[\gamma \mid \mathbf{y}]]$. So minimizing the expected posterior loss shares the same mathematics as A-optimality. For the normal model (1.7) with a conjugate (i.e., normal) prior for the vector $\boldsymbol{\mu}$, the D- and E-optimality criteria defined in Section 1.6 applied to $E[Var[\gamma \mid \mathbf{y}]]$ also find a decision-theoretic justification (see Giovagnoli and Verdinelli (1983) and Pilz (1991)).

There are also other approaches tailored on the Bayesian outlook. When an experiment has "information" as its generic objective, the utility function can be based on a measure of information given by the experiment, typically Shannon's (Shannon, 1948). More precisely, the idea is to choose in a given class of experimental designs the one which maximizes the expectation of the difference between Shannon's information based on the posterior distribution of the parameters and that based on the prior (Lindley, 1956). It can be shown that it is equivalent to choosing the experimental plan that maximizes the expected Kullback-Leibler divergence between the posterior and the prior of the model parameters, i.e.,

$$\int \left\{ \int_{\Omega} \log \frac{p(\gamma \mid \mathbf{y})}{p(\gamma)} p(\gamma \mid \mathbf{y}) d\gamma \right\} f(\mathbf{y}) d\mathbf{y},$$

where $f(\mathbf{y}) = \int f(\mathbf{y} \mid \gamma) p(\gamma) d\gamma$ is the marginal distribution of the responses.

The purpose of the experiment may alternatively be prediction of future outcomes, often required in clinical applications or in quality control. A priori, the predictive distribution of the next observation is

$$f(y) = \int_{\Omega} f(y \mid \gamma) p(\gamma) d\gamma,$$

whereas a posteriori the predictive distribution is

$$f(y_{n+1} \mid y_1, \ldots, y_n) = \int_{\Omega} f(y_n + 1 \mid \gamma) p(\gamma \mid y_1, \ldots, y_n) d\gamma.$$

In this case, the choice of the experimental plan can be made evaluating the information contents of the prior and of the posterior predictive distributions and maximizing the expected gain in Shannon's information, which again is equivalent to considering the expectation of the Kullback-Leibler divergence of the posterior predictive from the prior predictive. Other authors (Eaton et al., 1996) consider minimizing quadratic measures of distance between the predictive distributions.

The problem of allocating v treatments sequentially when the experiment has a utilitarian purpose has been mentioned at the start of Chapter 4. In the Bayesian literature it is known as a *bandit problem* (Berry and Fridstedt, 1985). It consists of sequential selection of the observations from v stochastic processes (the *arms*), corresponding to the treatments. The classic objective is to choose a strategy that maximizes the expected value of a *payoff* function $\sum_n \alpha_n Y_n$, where Y_n is the response at stage n and α_n are non-negative numbers. Given a sequence $\{\alpha_1, \alpha_2, \ldots, \alpha_n, \ldots\}$, the payoff is averaged over the unknown parameters with respect to some prior distribution quantifying the knowledge of the experimenter concerning the v arms. With a finite sequence $\{\alpha_1, \alpha_2, \ldots, \alpha_n\}$, to solve this sequential decision problem one must start from the last stage and work backwards (this is properly explained for instance in Bernardo and Smith (1994)), and solve a problem in dynamic programming. Practical implementation of this, however, is in general prohibitive. In some cases the authors choose designs with only a very limited number of stages, for instance two stages.

A multipurpose approach proposed by Verdinelli and Kadane (1992) combines inference on γ with the gain given by the value of the response $\mathbf{y}$, in the same spirit as the compound criteria introduced in Chapter 5 of the present book. The authors suggest a utility function which is a linear combination of the total expected value of future observations and the Shannon's information of the experiment:

$$U = \int \left\{ \mathbf{y}^t \mathbf{1} + \omega \left[\int_{\Omega} p(\gamma|\mathbf{y}) \log p(\gamma|\mathbf{y}) d\gamma \right] \right\} f(\mathbf{y}) d\mathbf{y},$$

where ω is a weight that measures the relative contribution of the two components. When the purpose is both prediction and parameter estimation, Verdinelli (1992) suggests a utility function obtained as a convex combination of the relative utilities.

We now give a simple example of a Bayesian design for comparing v treatments under a linear model with normality assumptions:

Example B.1 *Let the model be (1.7) with known variances σ_j^2 and assume a conjugate normal prior for the vector $\boldsymbol{\mu}$ of the treatment effects, with the prior covariance matrix $\mathbf{D}$ of $\boldsymbol{\mu}$ known. Then the posterior covariance matrix after n_j observations of treatment j ($j = 1, \ldots, v$) is*

$$\mathbf{V} = \left(\left[diag \left(\frac{\sigma_j^2}{n_j} \right)_{j=1,\ldots,v} \right]^{-1} + \mathbf{D}^{-1} \right)^{-1}.$$

This is true regardless of whether the posterior has been updated after each observation or just at the end. It is often reasonable to assume that the treatment effects are a priori uncorrelated, so that $\mathbf{D} = diag\left(\tau_j^2\right)_{j=1,\ldots,v}$; different values of τ_j reflect different degrees of prior uncertainty on the parameters, which might be realistic, especially with a control treatment. If the loss W is taken to be quadratic, the Bayesian A-optimal design is

$$n_k = \frac{\sigma_k}{\sum_j \sigma_j} \left(n + \sum_{j=1}^{v} \frac{\sigma_j^2}{\tau_j^2} \right) - \frac{\sigma_k^2}{\tau_k^2}, \qquad \forall k = 1, \ldots, v \tag{B.2}$$

(assuming that the quantities (B.2) are all ≥ 0). The intuitive interpretation is that the prior information is the equivalent of $m_k = (\sigma_k/\tau_k)^2$ previous observations on treatment k ($k = 1, \ldots, v$) and the optimal allocation is Neyman's (see Table 1.1) out of a total number $n + \sum_{j=1}^{v} m_j$ observations. Clearly when the prior information on some treatment is vague, i.e., $\tau_k^2 \to \infty$, this is exactly the same as the Neyman allocation for model (1.7). On the other hand, the treatments for which τ_k^2 is very small will not be observed.

For fixed sample size n and known σ_j's, the example just shown gives a fixed optimum target allocation of the treatments. When the σ_j's are unknown, Verdinelli (2000) has shown that, for the most common choices of optimal design criteria, Bayesian experimental designs are, at worst, only mildly affected by the knowledge of data variability.

The above example is straightforward because the model is linear. With non-linear models a rigorous, i.e., fully Bayesian, approach often leads to a mathematically very complex problem. As previously mentioned, a widespread viewpoint is to combine a Bayesian perspective on the design with a frequentist one on the statistical analysis of the data, giving rise to a hybrid approach. Going back to Chaloner and Larntz (1989), the following methods are practiced. They are sometimes described as "probability only" approaches, since they do not specify a utility or loss function.

Method 1: The loss of information is measured by a frequentist criterion, as in Section 1.6. This criterion will be a function of Fisher's information matrix and in general will depend on the unknown parameters. If a prior distribution on the parameters is available, the criterion's expectation is calculated and then minimized over the set of all possible target allocations.

Method 2: Fisher's information matrix is averaged over the parameter prior, and a target allocation is chosen that optimizes a suitable function of it. This alternative procedure is less convincing in terms of a theoretical justification.

Method 3: When the target, obtained by an optimal frequentist design criterion or otherwise, depends on the unknown parameters, it is averaged over the parameter prior.

Method 4: The statistical model is averaged with respect to the parameter prior and a target allocation is calculated.

These ad hoc approaches may turn out to be fairly efficient in particular instances, but it would be an arbitrary judgment to claim that they are "optimal" in any sense, apart perhaps from Method 1.

Bayesian adaptive experimental designs

All the above methods give rise to a known target allocation, and the treatments can be assigned to the units in a non-adaptive way so as to achieve the desired target. If the target allocation is known prior to the beginning of the experiment, there is no apparent need to plan the experiment sequentially. The need may arise, though, in order to introduce a randomization component; if so, the allocation-adaptive procedures of Chapter 2 can be applied within a Bayesian context too. Some designs get labeled as Bayesian just because a target allocation obtained by Bayesian arguments is used as the allocation probability; Atkinson (2002) and Atkinson and Biswas (2005b) describe some designs as Bayesian Biased Coin ones, due to the fact that the allocation targets (one is non-skewed and the other is skewed) were obtained by a Bayesian approach due to Ball et al. (1993), that combines two utility functions, one for inferential precision and one for randomness.

To target an allocation which depends on the parameters, an appealing alternative is to use the data to update the posterior distribution of the treatment effects at each stage, rather than rely on the prior throughout the experiment. The four hybrid Bayesian-frequentist methods listed above for non-sequential experiments get practiced in sequential contexts too. This also enables use of the accrued information to redress the allocation towards the most promising treatments. Thus, in some circumstances the whole apparatus of response-adaptive treatment allocation discussed in some chapters of this book works for Bayesian experiments too.

Reiterating Method 1 is fairly common; it is used for instance by Haines et al. (2003). An example of reiterated Method 3 is the *continual reassessment* by O'Quigley et al. (1990) and subsequent modifications thereof, for targeting an unknown quantile. Reiterated Method 4 is used for instance by Yin and Yuan (2011).

With binary outcomes, given two treatments A and B with probabilities of success p_A and p_B, a suitable Bayesian ethical target for A might be $\Pr(p_A > p_B)$. An idea that goes back a long time (Thompson, 1933) is to use the posterior probability $\Pr(p_A > p_B \mid \mathbf{y})$, as the allocation mechanism of the experimental units. We may start with the same Beta distribution $Beta(a, b)$ as our prior for both p_A and p_B, with p_A and p_B a priori independent. Having observed s_j successes out of n_j assignments on treatment j ($j = A, B$), the *posterior* on p_j is also Beta with $Beta(a + s_A, b + n_j - s_j)$. Then, $\Pr(p_A > p_B \mid \mathbf{y})$ is our allocation probability for A at the next step. It is interesting to point out that the Bayesian approach is conditional on the design, and if p_A and p_B are a priori independent, they will continue to be (conditionally) independent also a posteriori.

To avoid undesirable variability, it is common practice to consider a stabilizing transformation, namely to take the allocation probabilities of treatment A proportional to $\Pr(p_A > p_B \mid \mathbf{y})^v$ and vice versa for B, where v is a positive quantity that modulates the tradeoff between the exploration and the exploitation aims of the experiment: $v = 1/2$ is the recommended value, based on empirical experience (Thall and Wathen, 2007). Extensions of the theory include a predictive criterion for selecting v that also allows its progressive reassessment based on interim analysis data, and the so-called *randomized probability matching*, a multi-armed bandit that randomly allocates observations to arms according the Bayesian posterior probability that each arm is the best.

The Bayesian procedures described so far refer to fixed sample size n, whereas often the problem is finding an optimal n, for instance to guarantee a given threshold for the power of a test under the alternative hypothesis. Since the seminal paper on this topic by Adcock (1997), the research on optimal sample size in a Bayesian framework has grown steadily. In Bayesian inference, often the Bayes factor is utilized as the criterion to choose between two hypotheses and the sample size problem is embedded in this context. Clinical applications are privileged: De Santis et al. (2004), followed by Mlan et al. (2006), were the first to systematically consider Bayesian sample size problems for case-control studies, and a related article is, for instance, Gubbiotti and De Santis (2011).

Bibliography

C. J. Adcock. Sample size determination: a review. *The Statistician*, 46:261–283, 1997.

G. Aletti, C. May, and P. Secchi. A central limit theorem and related results for a two-color randomly reinforced urn. *Advances in Applied Probability*, 41(3):829 –844, 2009.

G. Aletti, A. Ghiglietti, and A. M. Paganoni. A modified randomly reinforced urn design. *Journal of Applied Probability*, 50(2):486–498, 2013.

K. B. Athreya and S. Karlin. Embedding of urn schemes into continuous time Markov branching processes and related limit theorems. *Annals of Mathematical Statistics*, 39:1801–1817, 1968.

A. C. Atkinson. Optimum biased-coin designs for sequential clinical trials with prognostic factors. *Biometrika*, 69:61–67, 1982.

A. C. Atkinson. Optimum biased-coin designs for sequential treatment allocation with covariate information. *Statistics in Medicine*, 18:1741–1752, 1999.

A. C. Atkinson. The comparison of designs for sequential clinical trials with covariate information. *Journal of the Royal Statistical Society Series A*, 165:349–373, 2002.

A. C. Atkinson. Bias and loss: the two sides of a biased coin. *Statistics in Medicine*, 31:3494–3503, 2012.

A. C. Atkinson. Selecting a biased-coin design. *Statistical Science*, 29(1):144–163, 2014.

A. C. Atkinson and A. Biswas. Adaptive biased-coin designs for skewing the allocation proportion in clinical trials with normal responses. *Statistics in Medicine*, 24: 2477–2492, 2005a.

A. C. Atkinson and A. Biswas. Bayesian adaptive biased-coin designs for clinical trials with normal responses. *Biometrics*, 61:118–125, 2005b.

A. C. Atkinson and A. Biswas. *Randomised Response-Adaptive Designs in Clinical Trials*. Boca Raton: Chapman & Hall/CRC Press, 2014.

A. C. Atkinson and V. V. Fedorov. The design of experiments for discriminating between two rival models. *Biometrika*, 62(1):57–70, 1975a.

A. C. Atkinson and V. V. Fedorov. Optimal design: experiments for discriminating between several models. *Biometrika*, 62(2):289–303, 1975b.

A. C. Atkinson, A. N. Donev, and R. Tobias. *Optimum Experimental Designs, with SAS*. Oxford University Press, 2007.

A. C. Atkinson, A. Biswas, and L. Pronzato. Covariate-balanced response-adaptive designs for clinical trials with continuous responses that target allocation probabilities. *Technical Report NI11042-DAE, Isaac Newton Institute for Mathematical Sciences, Cambridge*, 2011.

D. Azriel, M. Mandel, and Y. Rinott. Optimal allocation to maximize power of two-sample tests for binary response. *Biometrika*, 99:101–113, 2012.

J. S. Babb and A. Rogatko. Patient specific dosing in a cancer Phase I clinical trial. *Statistics in Medicine*, 20:2079–2090, 2001.

Z. D. Bai and F. Hu. Asymptotics in randomized urn models. *The Annals of Applied Probability*, 15:914–940, 2005.

Z. D. Bai, F. Hu, and W. F. Rosenberger. Asymptotic properties of adaptive designs with delayed responses. *The Annals of Statistics*, 30:122–139, 2002a.

Z. D. Bai, F. Hu, and L.-X. Zhang. Gaussian approximation theorems for urn models and their applications. *The Annals of Applied Probability*, 12(4):1149–1173, 2002b.

R. A. Bailey and P. R. Nelson. Hadamard randomization: a valid restriction of random permuted blocks. *Biometrical Journal*, 45(5):554–560, 2003.

S. Balaji, H. M. Mahmoud, and O. Watanabe. Distributions in the Ehrenfest process. *Statistics and Probability Letters*, 76(7):666–674, 2006.

A. Baldi Antognini. On the speed of convergence of some urn designs for the balanced allocation of two treatments. *Metrika*, 62(2):309–322, 2005.

A. Baldi Antognini. A theoretical analysis of the power of biased-coin designs. *Journal of Statistical Planning and Inference*, 138:1792–1798, 2008.

A. Baldi Antognini and I. Crimaldi. A dose-finding sequential method for targeting a given mean response: Up & Down experiments. In *Atti della XLIII Riunione Scientifica della Societá Italiana di Statistica, Torino, 14-16 giugno 2006*, pages 415–426, 2006.

A. Baldi Antognini and S. Giannerini. Generalized Pólya urn designs with null balance. *Journal of Applied Probability*, 44:661–669, 2007.

A. Baldi Antognini and A. Giovagnoli. A new "biased-coin design" for the sequential allocation of two treatments. *Journal of the Royal Statistical Society Series C*, 53: 651–664, 2004.

A. Baldi Antognini and A. Giovagnoli. On the large sample optimality of sequential designs for comparing two or more treatments. *Sequential Analysis*, 24:205–217, 2005.

A. Baldi Antognini and A. Giovagnoli. On the asymptotic inference for response-adaptive experiments. *Metron*, LXIV(1):29–45, 2006.

A. Baldi Antognini and A. Giovagnoli. Compound optimal allocation for individual and collective ethics in binary clinical trials. *Biometrika*, 97:935–946, 2010.

A. Baldi Antognini and M. Zagoraiou. The covariate-adaptive biased coin design for balancing clinical trials in the presence of prognostic factors. *Biometrika*, 98: 519–535, 2011.

A. Baldi Antognini and M. Zagoraiou. Multi-objective optimal designs in comparative clinical trials with covariates: the reinforced doubly-adaptive biased coin design. *The Annals of Statistics*, 40:1315–1345, 2012.

A. Baldi Antognini and M. Zagoraiou. On the almost sure convergence of adaptive allocation procedures. *Bernoulli*, to appear:(available online), 2015.

A. Baldi Antognini, P. Bortot, and A. Giovagnoli. Randomized group up and down experiments. *Annals of the Institute of Statistical Mathematics*, 60:45–59, 2008.

A. Baldi Antognini, A. Giovagnoli, and M. Zagoraiou. Some recent developments in the design of adaptive clinical trials. *Statistica*, 72(4):375–393, 2012.

F. G. Ball, A. F. M. Smith, and I. Verdinelli. Biased coin design with a Bayesian bias. *Journal of Statistical Planning and Inference*, 34:403–421, 1993.

U. Bandyopadhyay and R. Bhattacharya. An urn based covariate adjusted response adaptive allocation design. *Statistical Methods in Medical Research*, 21(2):135–148, 2012.

U. Bandyopadhyay and A. Biswas. Some sequential tests in clinical trials based on randomized play-the-winner rule. *Calcutta Statistical Association Bulletin*, 47: 67–89, 1997a.

U. Bandyopadhyay and A. Biswas. Sequential comparison of two treatments in clinical trials: a decision theoretic approach based on randomized play-the-winner rule. *Sequential Analysis*, 16:66–92, 1997b.

U. Bandyopadhyay and A. Biswas. Some sequential-type conditional tests in clinical trials based on generalized randomized play-the-winner rule. *Metron*, LVIII:187–200, 2000.

U. Bandyopadhyay and A. Biswas. Adaptive designs for normal responses with prognostic factors. *Biometrika*, 88:409–419, 2001.

U. Bandyopadhyay and A. Biswas. Test of Bernoulli success probability in inverse sampling for nearer alternatives using adaptive allocation. *Statistica Neerlandica*, 56(4):387–399, 2002.

U. Bandyopadhyay and A. Biswas. Non-parametric group sequential designs in randomized clinical trials. *Australian and New Zealand Journal of Statistics*, 45: 367–376, 2003.

U. Bandyopadhyay, A. Biswas, and R. Bhattacharya. Adaptive designs for normal responses with prognostic factors. *Statistics in Medicine*, 26:4386–4399, 2007.

U. Bandyopadhyay, A. Biswas, and R. Bhattacharya. Drop-the-loser design in the presence of covariates. *Metrika*, 67:1–15, 2009.

Y. Barbachano, D. S. Coad, and D. R. Robinson. Predictability of designs which adjust for imbalances in prognostic factors. *Journal of Statistical Planning and Inference*, 138:756–767, 2008.

G. A. Barnard. Discussion of paper by J. Kiefer. *Journal of the Royal Statistical Society Series B*, 21:311–312, 1959.

R. H. Bartlett, D. W. Roloff, R. G. Cornell, A. F. Andrews, P. W. Dillon, and J. B. Zwischenberger. Extracorporeal circulation in neonatal respiratory failure: A prospective randomized study. *Pediatrics*, 6:479–487, 1985.

C. B. Begg and B. Iglewicz. A treatment allocation procedure for sequential clinical trials. *Biometrics*, 36:81–90, 1980.

A. W. Beggs. On the convergence of reinforcement learning. *Journal of Economic Theory*, 122:1–36, 2005.

V. W. Berger. A review of methods for ensuring the comparability of comparison groups in randomized clinical trials. *Reviews on Recent Clinical Trials*, 1:81– 86, 2006.

V. W. Berger, A. Ivanova, and M. D. Knoll. Minimizing predictability while retaining balance through the use of less restrictive randomization procedures. *Statistics in Medicine*, 22:3017–3028, 2003.

J. M. Bernardo and A. F. M. Smith. *Bayesian Theory*. Wiley, New York, 1994.

D. A. Berry. Bayesian statistics and the efficiency and ethics of clinical trials. *Statistical Science*, 19(1):175–187, 2004.

D. A. Berry. Adaptive clinical trials: the promise and the caution. *Journal of Clinical Oncology*, 29(6):606–609, 2011.

D. A. Berry and B. Fridstedt. *Bandit Problems: Sequential Allocation of Experiments*. Chapman & Hall, London, 1985.

D. A. Berry and M. Sobel. An improved procedure for selecting the better of two Bernoulli populations. *Journal of the American Statistical Association*, 68:979–984, 1973.

S. M. Berry, B. P. Carlin, J. J. Lee, and P. Muller. *Bayesian Adaptive Methods for Clinical Trials*. Chapman & Hall/CRC Biostatistics Series, 2011.

A. Biswas and R. Bhattacharya. Treatment adaptive allocations in randomized clinical trials: An overview. In Annpey Pong and Shein-Chung Chow, editors, *Handbook of Adaptive Designs in Pharmaceutical and Clinical Development*, pages 17:1–17:19, Boca Raton, 2011. Chapman & Hall.

A. Biswas and S. Mandal. Optimal three-treatment response-adaptive designs for Phase III clinical trials with binary responses. In Jesus Lopez-Fidalgo, Juan Manuel Rodriguez-Diaz, and Ben Torsney, editors, *mODa 8- Advances in Model-Oriented Design and Analysis, Contributions to Statistics*, pages 33–40, Heidelberg, 2007. Physica-Verlag.

A. Biswas, H. H. Huang, and W. T. Huang. Covariate-adjusted adaptive designs for continuous responses in a Phase III clinical trial: recommendation for practice. *Journal of Biopharmaceutical Statistics*, 16:227–239, 2006.

A. Biswas, S. Mandal, and R. Bhattacharya. Multi-treatment optimal response-adaptive designs for Phase III clinical trials. *Journal of Korean Statistical Society*, 40:33–44, 2011.

D. H. Blackwell and J. L. Hodges. Design for the control of selection bias. *Annals of Mathematical Statistics*, 28:449–460, 1957.

P. Bortot and A. Giovagnoli. Up-and-down experiments of first and second order. *Journal of Statistical Planning and Inference*, 134(1):236–253, 2005.

S. Boyd and L. Vandenberghe. *Convex Optimization*. Cambridge University Press, Cambridge, 2004.

C. F. Burman. *On Sequential Treatment Allocations in Clinical Trials*. PhD Dissertation. Department of Mathematics. Goteborg University, 1996.

B. P. Carlin and T. A. Louis. *Bayesian Methods for Data Analysis, Third Edition*. Boca Raton: Chapman & Hall/CRC Press, 2009.

K. Chaloner and K. Larntz. Optimal Bayesian design applied to logistic experiments. *Journal of Statistical Planning and Inference*, 18:181–208, 1989.

K. Chaloner and I. Verdinelli. Bayesian optimal design: a review. *Statistical Science*, 10(3):273–304, 1995.

P. Chaudhuri and P. A. Mykland. Nonlinear experiments: optimal design and inference based on likelihood. *Journal of the American Statistical Association*, 88: 538–546, 1993.

Y.-P. Chen. Biased coin design with imbalance tolerance. *Communications in Statistics. Stochastic Models*, 15:953–975, 1999.

Y.-P. Chen. Which design is better? Ehrenfest urn versus biased coin. *Advances in Applied Probability*, 32:738–749, 2000.

Y.-P. Chen. A central limit property under a modified Ehrenfest urn design. *Journal of Applied Probability*, 43(2):409–420, 2006.

CHMP. Reflection paper on methodological issues in confirmatory clinical trials planned with an adaptive design, 2007. Available online.

S. C. Chow and M. Chang. *Adaptive Design Methods in Clinical Trials*. Boca Raton: Chapman & Hall/CRC Press, 2007.

M. Clyde and K. Chaloner. The equivalence of constrained and weighted designs in multiple objective design problems. *Journal of the American Statistical Association*, 91:1236–1244, 1996.

D. S. Coad. Response adaptive randomization. In *Encyclopedia of Clinical Trials*, New York, 2008. John Wiley & Sons.

D. S. Coad and M. Woodroofe. Corrected confidence intervals for adaptive nonlinear regression models. *Journal of Statistical Planning and Inference*, 130:63–83, 2005.

D. Cook and W. Wong. On the equivalence of constrained and compound optimal designs. *Journal of the American Statistical Association*, 89:687–692, 1994.

D. R. Cox. *Principles of Statistical Inference*. Cambridge University Press, Cambridge, 2006.

D. R. Cox and D. V. Hinkley. *Theoretical Statistics*. London: Chapman & Hall; New York: Halsted Press, 1974.

W. G. Cumberland and R. M. Royall. Does simple random sampling provide adequate balance? *Journal of Royal Statistical Society Series B*, 50:118–124, 1988.

F. De Santis, M. Perone Pacifico, and V. Sambucini. Optimal predictive sample size for case-control studies. *Journal of the Royal Statistical Society Series C*, 53(3): 427–441, 2004.

C. Derman. Non-parametric up-and-down experimentation. *Annals of Mathematical Statistics*, 28:795–799, 1957.

H. Dette. On a generalization of the Ehrenfest urn model. *Journal of Applied Probability*, 31:930–939, 1994.

H. Dette. Designing experiments with respect to standardized optimality criteria. *Journal of the Royal Statistical Society Series B*, 59:97–110, 1997.

W. J. Dixon and A. M. Mood. A method for obtaining and analyzing sensitivity data. *Journal of the American Statistical Association*, 43:109–126, 1948.

V. Dragalin and V. V. Fedorov. Adaptive designs for dose-finding based on efficacy-toxicity response. *Journal of Statistical Planning and Inference*, 136:1800–1823, 2006.

S. D. Durham and N. Flournoy. Random walks for quantile estimation. *Statistical Decision Theory and Related Topics*, 43:467–476, 1994.

S. D. Durham and K. F. Yu. Randomized play-the leader rules for sequential sampling from two populations. *Probability in the Engineering and Informational Sciences*, 26:355–367, 1990.

S. D. Durham, N. Flournoy, and W. F. Rosenberger. Asymptotic normality of maximum likelihood estimators from multiparameter response-driven designs. *Journal of Statistical Planning and Inference*, 60:69–76, 1997.

M. L. Eaton, A. Giovagnoli, and P. Sebastiani. A predictive approach to the Bayesian design problem with application to the normal regression models. *Biometrika*, 83 (1):111–125, 1996.

B. Efron. Forcing sequential experiments to be balanced. *Biometrika*, 58:403–417, 1971.

B. Efron. Randomizing and balancing a complicated sequential experiment. In R. G. Miller, B. Efron, B. W. Brown, and L. E. Moses, editors, *Biostatistics Casebook*, pages 19–30, New York, 1980. John Wiley & Sons.

J. R. Eisele. The doubly adaptive biased coin design for sequential clinical trials. *Journal of Statistical Planning and Inference*, 38:249–62, 1994.

J. R. Eisele and M. Woodroofe. Central limit theorems for doubly adaptive biased coin designs. *The Annals of Statistics*, 23:234–254, 1995.

G. Elfving. Optimum allocation in linear regression theory. *The Annals of Mathematical Statistics*, 23(2):255–262, 1952.

R. Etzioni and J. B. Kadane. Optimal experimental design for another's analysis. *Journal of the American Statistical Association*, 88(424):1404–1411, 1993.

FDA. Guidance for industry. adaptive design clinical trials for drugs and biologics (draft document), 2010. URL `http://www.fda.gov/downloads/Drugs/Guidances/ucm201790.pdf`. Available online.

V. V. Fedorov. *Theory of Optimal Experiments*. Academic Press, New York, 1972.

P. Flajolet, J. Gabarró, and H. Pekari. Analytic urns. *The Annals of Probability*, 33 (3):1200–1233, 2005.

P. Flajolet, P. Dumas, and V. Puyhaubert. Some exactly solvable models of urn process theory. In *DMTCS Proceedings of the Fourth Colloquium on Mathematics and Computer Science Algorithms, Trees, Combinatorics and Probabilities*, pages 59–118, Nancy, France, 2006.

N. Flournoy, C. May, and P. Secchi. Asymptotically optimal response-adaptive designs for allocating the best treatment: an overview. *International Statistical Review*, 80(2):293–305, 2012.

B. Friedman. A simple urn model. *Communications on Pure and Applied Mathematics*, 2:59–70, 1949.

M. Fushimi. An improved version of a Sobel-Weiss play-the-winner procedure for selecting the better of two binomial populations. *Biometrika*, 60:517–523, 1973.

M. Geraldes, V. Melfi, C. Page, and H. Zhang. The doubly adaptive weighted difference design. *Journal of Statistical Planning and Inference*, 136:1923–1939, 2006.

M. Gezmu and N. Flournoy. Group up-and-down designs for dose-finding. *Journal of Statistical Planning and Inference*, 136:1749–1764, 2006.

A. Giovagnoli. Markovian properties of some biased coin designs. In A. Di Bucchianico, H. Läuter, and H.P. Wynn, editors, *mODa 7-Advances in Model-Oriented Design Analysis, Contributions to Statistics*, pages 69–76, Heidelberg, 2004. Physica-Verlag.

A. Giovagnoli and N. Pintacuda. Properties of frequency distributions induced by general 'up-and-down' methods for estimating quantiles. *Journal of Statistical Planning and Inference*, 74:51–63, 1998.

A. Giovagnoli and I. Verdinelli. Bayes D-optimal and E-optimal block designs. *Biometrika*, 70:695–706, 1983.

A. Giovagnoli, F. Pukelsheim, and H. P. Wynn. Group-invariant orderings and experimental designs. *Journal of Statistical Planning and Inference*, 17(2):159–171, 1987.

R. Gouet. Martingale functional central limit theorems for a generalized Pólya urn. *The Annals of Probability*, 21(3):1624–1639, 1993.

S. Gubbiotti and F. De Santis. A Bayesian method for the choice of the sample size in equivalence trials. *Australian and New Zealand Journal of Statistics*, 53:443–460, 2011.

E. T. Gwise, J. Hu, and F. Hu. Optimal biased coins for two-arm clinical trials. *Statistics and Its Interface*, 1:125–135, 2008.

L. M. Haines, I. Perevozskaya, and W. F. Rosenberger. Bayesian optimal design for Phase I clinical trials. *Biometrics*, 59:591–600, 2003.

J. B. S. Haldane. On a method of estimating frequencies. *Biometrika*, 33:222–225, 1945.

B. Han, N. H. Enas, and D. McEntegart. Randomization by minimization for unbalanced treatment allocation. *Statistics in Medicine*, 28:3329–3346, 2009.

D. L. Hawkins. A proof of the asymptotic normality of the inverse sampling estimator in finite population sampling. *Journal of Statistical Planning and Inference*, 92: 175–180, 2001.

S. Heritier, V. Gebski, and A. Pillai. Dynamic balancing randomization in controlled clinical trials. *Statistics in Medicine*, 24:3729–3741, 2005.

I. Higueras, J. Moler, F. Plo, and M. San Miguel. Urn models and differential algebraic equations. *Journal of Applied Probability*, 40(2):401–412, 2003.

I. Higueras, J. Moler, F. Plo, and M. San Miguel. Central limit theorems for generalized Pólya urn models. *Journal of Applied Probability*, 43(4):938–951, 2006.

D. G. Hoel. An inverse stopping rule for play-the-winner sampling. *Journal of the American Statistical Association*, 67:148–151, 1972.

P. G. Hoel, S. C. Port, and C. J. Stone. *Introduction to Stochastic Processes.* Houghton Mifflin Company, Boston, 1972.

N. Holford, S. C. Ma, and B. A. Ploeger. Clinical trial simulation: A review. *Clinical Pharmacology and Therapeutics*, 88:166–182, 2010.

F. Hu and W. F. Rosenberger. Optimality, variability, power: evaluating response-adaptive randomization procedures for treatment comparisons. *Journal of the American Statistical Association*, 98:671–678, 2003.

F. Hu and W. F. Rosenberger. *The Theory of Response-Adaptive Randomization in Clinical Trials.* New York: John Wiley & Sons, 2006.

F. Hu and L.-X. Zhang. Asymptotic properties of doubly adaptive biased coin designs for multi-treatment clinical trials. *The Annals of Statistics*, 32:268–301, 2004.

F. Hu, W. F. Rosenberger, and L.-X. Zhang. Asymptotically best response-adaptive randomization procedures. *Journal of Statistical Planning and Inference*, 136: 1911–1922, 2006.

F. Hu, L.-X. Zhang, S. H. Cheung, and W. S. Chan. Doubly adaptive biased coin designs with delayed responses. *The Canadian Journal of Statistics*, 36:541–559, 2008.

F. Hu, L.-X. Zhang, and X. He. Efficient randomized adaptive designs. *The Annals of Statistics*, 37:2543–2560, 2009.

Y. Hu and F. Hu. Asymptotic properties of covariate-adaptive randomization. *The Annals of Statistics*, 40:1794–1815, 2012.

K. Inoue and S. Aki. Pólya urn models under general replacement schemes. *Journal of the Japan Statistical Society*, 31(2):193–205, 2001.

A. Ivanova. A play-the-winner type urn model with reduced variability. *Metrika*, 58: 1–13, 2003a.

A. Ivanova. A new dose-finding design for bivariate outcomes. *Biometrics*, 59: 1003–1009, 2003b.

A. Ivanova and N. Flournoy. A birth and death urn for ternary outcomes: stochastic processes applied to urn models. In C. A. Charalambides, M. V. Koutras, and N. Balakrishnan, editors, *Probability and Statistical Models with Applications*, pages 583–560, Boca Raton, 2001. Chapman & Hall.

A. Ivanova and N. Flournoy. Up-and-down designs in toxicity studies. In S. Chevret, editor, *Statistical Methods for Dose-finding Experiments*, pages 115–130, Chichester, 2006. John Wiley & Sons.

A. Ivanova and K. Wang. Bivariate isotonic design for dose-finding with ordered groups. *Statistics in Medicine*, 25:2018–2026, 2006.

A. Ivanova, W. F. Rosenberger, S. D. Durham, and N. Flournoy. A birth and death urn for randomized clinical trials: asymptotic methods. *Sankhyá series B*, 62:104–118, 2000.

A. Ivanova, A. Montazer-Haghighi, S. G. Mohant, and S. D. Durham. Improved up-and-down designs for Phase I trials. *Statistics in Medicine*, 22(2):69–82, 2003.

S. Janson. Functional limit theorems for multitype branching processes and generalized Pólya urns. *Stochastic Process and their Applications*, 110(2):177–245, 2004.

C. Jennison and B. W. Turnbull. *Group Sequential Methods with Applications to Clinical Trials.* Chapman & Hall, New York, 2000.

C. Jennison and B. W. Turnbull. Group sequential tests with outcome-dependent treatment assignment. *Sequential Analysis*, 20(4):209–234, 2001.

Y. Jeon and F. Hu. Optimal adaptive designs for binary response trials with three treatments. *Statistics in Biopharmaceutical Research*, 2:310–318, 2010.

N. L. Johnson and S. Kotz. *Urn Models and their Application.* John Wiley & Sons, New York, 1977.

L. D. Kaiser. Inefficiency of randomization methods that balance on stratum margins and improvements with permuted blocks and sequential method. *Statistics in Medicine*, 31:1699–1706, 2012.

J. E. Kiefer and G. H. Weiss. Truncated version of a play-the-winner rule for choosing the better of two binomial populations. *Journal of the American Statistical Association*, 71:538 –546, 1974.

H. C. Kimko and S. B. Duffull. *Simulation for Designing Clinical Trials. A Pharmacokinetic-Pharmacodynamic Modeling Perspective*. Marcel Dekker, New York, 2003.

J. H. Klotz. Maximum entropy constrained balance randomization for clinical trials. *Biometrics*, 34:283–287, 1978.

E. L. Korn and B. Freidlin. Outcome-adaptive randomization: is it useful? *Journal of Clinical Oncology*, 29:771–776, 2011.

E. L. Korn, D. Midthune, T. T. Chen, L. V. Rubistein, M. C. Christian, and R. M. Simon. A comparison of two Phase I trial designs. *Statistics in Medicine*, 13: 1799–1806, 1994.

S. Kotz, H. Mahmoud, and P. Robert. On generalized Pólya urn models. *Statistics and Probability Letters*, 49(2):163–173, 2000.

A. Krause. The virtual patient: Developing drugs using modeling and simulation. *Chance*, 23:48–52, 2010.

O. M. Kuznetsova and Y. Tymofyeyev. Brick tunnel randomization for unequal allocation to two or more treatment groups. *Statistics in Medicine*, 30:812–824, 2011.

O. M. Kuznetsova and Y. Tymofyeyev. Preserving the allocation ratio at every allocation with biased coin randomization and minimization in studies with unequal allocation. *Statistics in Medicine*, 31:701–723, 2012.

J. M. Lachin. A review of methods for futility stopping based on conditional power. *Statistics in Medicine*, 24:2747–2764, 2005.

W. Li, S. D. Durham, and N. Flournoy. Randomized Pòlya urn designs. In *Proceedings of the Biometric Section, Chicago 1996*, pages 166–170, Alexandria, VA, 1997. American Statistical Association.

D. V. Lindley. On the measure of information provided by an experiment. *Annals of Statistics*, 27:986–1005, 1956.

D. V. Lindley. *Bayesian Statistics: A Review*. SIAM, Philadelphia, 1972.

J. K. Lindsey. *Parametrical Statistical Inference*. Oxford Science Publications, 1996.

R. J. A. Little and D. B. Rubin. *Statistical Analysis with Missing Data*. Wiley Series in Probability and Statistics, 2002.

J. Lopez-Fidalgo, C. Tommasi, and P. C. Trandafir. An optimal experimental design criterion for discriminating between non-normal models. *Journal of the Royal Statistical Society Series B*, 69:231–242, 2007.

T. Markaryan and W. F. Rosenberger. Exact properties of Efron's biased coin randomization procedure. *The Annals of Statistics*, 38:1546–1567, 2010.

P. C. Matthews and W. F. Rosenberger. Variance in randomized play-the-winner clinical trials. *Statistics and Probability Letters*, 35:233–240, 1997.

J. P. Matts and J. M. Lachin. Properties of permuted-block randomization in clinical trials. *Controlled Clinical Trials*, 9:327–344, 1988.

C. May and N. Flournoy. Asymptotics in response-adaptive designs generated by a two-color, randomly reinforced urn. *The Annals of Statistics*, 37(2):1058–1078, 2009.

P. McCullagh. Discussion of professor bather's paper. *J. Roy. Statist. Soc. Ser. B*, 43: 286–287, 1981.

V. Melfi and C. Page. Estimation after adaptive allocation. *Journal of Statistical Planning and Inference*, 29:353–363, 2000.

V. Melfi, C. Page, and M. Geraldes. An adaptive randomized design with application to estimation. *Canadian Journal of Statistics*, 29:107–116, 2001.

C. E. Mlan, L. Joseph, and D. B. Wolfson. Bayesian sample size determination for case-control studies. *Journal of the American Statistical Association*, 101:760–771, 2006.

G. Molenberghs and M. Kenward. *Missing Data in Clinical Studies*. John Wiley & Sons, New York, 2007.

P. Muliere, A. M. Paganoni, and P. Secchi. A randomly reinforced urn. *Journal of Statistical Planning and Inference*, 136(6):1853–1874, 2006a.

P. Muliere, A. M. Paganoni, and P. Secchi. Randomly reinforced urns for clinical trials with continuous responses. In *Proceedings of the XLIII Scientific Meeting of the Italian Statistical Society*, pages 403–414. Cluep, Padova, 2006b.

J. Ning and X. Huang. Response-adaptive randomization for clinical trials with adjustment for covariate imbalance. *Statistics in Medicine*, 29:1761–1768, 2010.

E. Nordbrock. An improved play-the-winner sampling procedure for selecting the better of two binomial populations. *Journal of the American Statistical Association*, 71:137 –139, 1976.

P. C. O'Brien and T. R. Fleming. A multiple testing procedure for clinical trials. *Biometrics*, 35:549–556, 1979.

N. L. Oden and M. J. McIntosh. Exact moments and probabilities for Wei's urn randomization model. *Statistics and Probability Letters*, 76:1694–1700, 2006.

J. O. O'Quigley, M. Pepe, and L. Fisher. Continual reassessment method: a practical design for Phase I clinical trials in cancer. *Biometrics*, 46(1):33–48, 1990.

A. P. Oron and P. D. Hoff. The k-in-a-row up-and-down design, revisited. *Statistics in Medicine*, 28:1805–1820, 2009.

L. Piccinato. *Metodi per le Decisioni Statistiche, 2nd edition.* Springer-Verlag, 2009.

J. Pilz. *Bayesian Estimation and Experimental Design in Linear Regression Models.* John Wiley & Sons, New York, 1991.

S. J. Pocock. Group sequential methods in the design and analysis of clinical trials. *Biometrika*, 64:191–199, 1977.

S. J. Pocock and R. Simon. Sequential treatment assignment with balancing for prognostic factors in the controlled clinical trial. *Biometrics*, 31:103–115, 1975.

N. Pouyanne. Classification of large Pòlya-Eggenberger urns with regard to their asymptotics. In *2005 International Conference on Analysis of Algorithms*, pages 275–285 (electronic). Association of Discrete Mathematics & Theoretical Computer Science, Nancy, 2005.

L. Pronzato and A. Pazman. *Design of Experiments in Nonlinear Models.* Lecture Notes in Statistics 212. Springer, 2013.

F. Pukelsheim. *Optimal Design of Experiment.* SIAM, 2006.

H. Robbins, G. Simons, and N. Starr. A sequential analogue of the Behrens-Fisher problem. *Annals of Mathematical Statistics*, 38:1384–1391, 1967.

W. F. Rosenberger. New directions in adaptive designs. *Statistical Science*, 11:137–149, 1996.

W. F. Rosenberger and J. L. Lachin. *Randomization in Clinical Trials: Theory and Practice.* John Wiley & Sons, New York, 2002.

W. F. Rosenberger and T. N. Sriram. Estimation for an adaptive allocation design. *Journal of Statistical Planning and Inference*, 59:309–19, 1996.

W. F. Rosenberger and O. Sverdlov. Handling covariates in the design of clinical trials. *Statistical Science*, 23:404–419, 2008.

W. F. Rosenberger, N. Flournoy, and S. D. Durham. Asymptotic normality of maximum likelihood estimators from multiparameter response-driven designs. *Journal of Statistical Planning and Inference*, 60:69–76, 1997.

W. F. Rosenberger, N. Stallard, A. Ivanova, C. N. Harper, and M. L. Ricks. Optimal adaptive designs for binary response trials. *Biometrics*, 57:909–913, 2001a.

W. F. Rosenberger, A. N. Vidyashankar, and D. K. Agarwal. Covariate-adjusted response-adaptive designs for binary response. *Journal of Biopharmaceutical Statistics*, 11:227–236, 2001b.

S. Ross. *Stochastic Processes.* John Wiley & Sons, New York, 1996.

I. Salama, A. Ivanova, and B. Quaqish. Efficient generation of constrained block allocation sequences. *Statistics in Medicine*, 27:1421–1428, 2008.

H. J. A. Schouten. Adaptive biased urn randomization in small strata when blinding is impossible. *Biometrics*, 51:1529–1535, 1995.

C. E. Shannon. A mathematical theory of communication. *Bell System Technology Journal*, 27:379–423 and 623–656, 1948.

J. Shao, X. Yu, and B. Zhong. A theory for testing hypotheses under covariate-adaptive randomization. *Biometrika*, 97:347–360, 2010.

D. Siegmund. *Sequential Analysis: Tests and Confidence Intervals.* Springer, Heidelberg, 1985.

D. F. Signorini, O. Leung, R. J. Simes, E. Beller, and V. J. Gebski. Dynamic balanced randomization for clinical trials. *Statistics in Medicine*, 12:2343–2350, 1993.

S. D. Silvey. *Optimal Designs.* Chapman & Hall, London, 1980.

N. Simon and R. Simon. Adaptive enrichment designs for clinical trials. *Biostatistics*, 14:613–625, 2013.

P. J. Smith. Inverse sampling. In S. Kotz and N. L. Johnson, editors, *Encyclopedia of Statistical Sciences*, volume 6, pages 3693–3697, New York, 1982. John Wiley & Sons.

R. L. Smith. Properties of biased coin designs in sequential clinical trials. *The Annals of Statistics*, 12:1018–1034, 1984a.

R. L. Smith. Sequential treatment allocation using biased coin designs. *Journal of the Royal Statistical Society Series B*, 46:519–543, 1984b.

R. T. Smythe. Central limit theorems for urn models. *Stochastic Processes and their Applications*, 65(1):115–137, 1996.

J. F. Soares and C. F. J. Wu. Some restricted randomization rules in sequential designs. *Communications in Statistics. Theory and Methods.*, 12:2017–2034, 1983.

M. Sobel and G. H. Weiss. Play-the-winner rule and inverse sampling in selecting the better of two binomial populations. *Journal of the American Statistical Association*, 66:545–551, 1971.

D. J. Spiegelhalter, K. R. Abrams, and J. P. Myles. *Bayesian Approaches to Clinical Trials and Health-Care Evaluation.* John Wiley & Sons, 2004.

B. E. Storer. Phase I trials. In P. Armitage and T. Colton, editors, *Encyclopedia of Biostatistics, 2nd edition*, pages 3365–3370, New York, 2005. John Wiley & Sons.

M. Stylianou and N. Flournoy. Dose finding using the biased coin up-and-down design and isotonic regression. *Biometrics*, 58:171–177, 2002.

R. Sun, S. H. Cheung, and L.-X. Zhang. A generalized drop-the-loser rule for multi-treatment clinical trials. *Journal of Statistical Planning and Inference*, 137:2011–2023, 2007.

O. Sverdlov and W. F. Rosenberger. On recent advances in optimal allocation designs in clinical trials. *Journal of Statistical Theory and Practice*, 7(4):753–773, 2013a.

O. Sverdlov and W. F. Rosenberger. Randomization in clinical trials: can we eliminate bias? *Clinical Investigation*, 3(1):37–47, 2013b.

D. R. Taves. Minimization: a new method of assigning patients to treatment and control groups. *Journal of Clinical Pharmacy and Therapeutics*, 15:443–453, 1974.

D. W. Taylor and E. G. Bosch. CTS: a clinical trials simulator. *Statistics in Medicine*, 9:787–801, 1990.

P. F. Thall and J. K. Wathen. Practical Bayesian adaptive randomisation in clinical trials. *European Journal of Cancer*, 43:859–866, 2007.

W. R. Thompson. On the likelihood that one unknown probability exceeds another in view of the evidence of two samples. *Biometrika*, 25:285–294, 1933.

M. C. K. Tweedie. Statistical properties of inverse Gaussian distributions. *Annals of Mathematical Statistics*, 28:362–377, 1957.

Y. Tymofyeyev, W. F. Rosenberger, and F. Hu. Implementing optimal allocation in sequential binary response experiments. *Journal of the American Statistical Association*, 102:224–234, 2007.

I. Verdinelli. Advances in Bayesian experimental designs. In J.M. Bernardo et al, editor, *Bayesian Statistics 4*, pages 467–481, Oxford, 1992. Oxford University Press.

I. Verdinelli. A note on Bayesian design for the normal linear model with unknown error variance. *Biometrika*, 87(1):222–227, 2000.

I. Verdinelli and J. B. Kadane. Bayesian designs for maximizing information and outcome. *Journal of the American Statistical Association*, 87:510–515, 1992.

G. von Bekesy. A new audiometer. *Acta Otolaryngology*, 35:411–422, 1947.

A. Wald. On the efficient design of statistical investigation. *Annals of Mathematical Statistics*, 14:134–140, 1943.

A. Wald. *Sequential Analysis*. John Wiley & Sons, New York, 1947.

L. J. Wei. A class of designs for sequential clinical trials. *Journal of the American Statistical Association*, 72:382–386, 1977.

L. J. Wei. The adaptive biased coin design for sequential experiments. *The Annals of Statistics*, 6:92–100, 1978a.

L. J. Wei. An application of an urn model to the design of sequential controlled clinical trials. *Journal of the American Statistical Association*, 73:559–563, 1978b.

L. J. Wei. The generalized Pòlya's urn design for sequential medical trials. *The Annals of Statistics*, 7:291–296, 1979.

L. J. Wei and S. Durham. The randomized play-the-winner rule in medical trials. *Journal of the American Statistical Association*, 73:840–843, 1978.

L. J. Wei, R. T. Smythe, and R. L. Smiyh. k-treatment comparisons with restricted randomization rules in clinical trials. *The Annals of Statistics*, 14:265–274, 1986.

G. B. Wetherill, H. Chen, and R. B. Vasudeva. Sequential estimation of quantal response curves: a new method of estimation. *Biometrika*, 53:439–454, 1966.

J. Whitehead. *The Design and Analysis of Sequential Clinical Trials*. John Wiley & Sons, 1997.

W. K. Wong and W. Zhu. Optimum treatment allocation rules under a variance heterogeneity model. *Statistics in Medicine*, 27:4581–4595, 2008.

M. Woodroofe and D. S. Coad. Corrected confidence intervals after sequential testing with applications to survival analysis. *Biometrika*, 83:763–777, 1996.

C. F. J. Wu. Asymptotic inference from sequential design in a nonlinear situation. *Biometrika*, 72:553–558, 1985.

H. Wynn. Results in the theory and construction of D-optimum experimental designs. *Journal of the Royal Statistical Society Series B*, 34:133–147, 1972.

G. Yin and Y. Yuan. Bayesian approach for adaptive design. In Annpey Pong and Shein-Chung Chow, editors, *Handbook of Adaptive Designs in Pharmaceutical and Clinical Development*, pages 3:1–3:19, Boca Raton, 2011. Chapman & Hall.

Y. Yuan, X. Huang, and S. Liu. A Bayesian response-adaptive covariate-balanced randomization design with application to a leukemia clinical trial. *Statistics in Medicine*, 30:1218–1229, 2011.

M. Zelen. Play-the-winner rule and the controlled clinical trials. *Journal of the American Statistical Association*, 64:131–146, 1969.

M. Zelen. The randomization and stratification of patients to clinical trials. *Journal of Chronic Diseases*, 27:365–375, 1974.

L. X. Zhang and F. Hu. A new family of covariate-adjusted response adaptive designs and their properties. *Applied Mathematics. A Journal of the Chinese Universities*, 24:1–13, 2009.

L.-X. Zhang and W. F. Rosenberger. Response-adaptive randomization for clinical trials with continuous outcomes. *Biometrics*, 62:562–569, 2006.

L.-X. Zhang, F. Hu, and S. H. Cheung. Asymptotic theorems of sequential estimation-adjusted urn models. *The Annals of Applied Probability*, 16(1):340–369, 2006.

L.-X. Zhang, W. S. Chan, S. H. Cheung, and F. Hu. A generalized drop-the-loser urn for clinical trials with delayed responses. *Statistica Sinica*, 17:387–409, 2007a.

L.-X. Zhang, F. Hu, S. H. Cheung, and W. S. Chan. Asymptotic properties of covariate-adjusted response-adaptive designs. *The Annals of Statistics*, 35:1166–1182, 2007b.

W. Zhao and Y. Weng. A simplified formula for quantification of the probability of deterministic assignments in permuted block randomization. *Journal of Statistical Planning and Inference*, 141(1):474–478, 2011a.

W. Zhao and Y. Weng. Block urn designs. a new randomization algorithm for sequential trials with two or more treatments and balanced or unbalanced allocation. *Contemporary Clinical Trials*, 32(1):953–96, 2011b.

W. Zhao, Y. Weng, Q. Wu, and Y. Palesch. Quantitative comparison of randomization designs in sequential clinical trials based on treatment balance and allocation randomness. *Pharmaceutical Statistics*, 11:39–48, 2012.

H. Zhu and F. Hu. Sequential monitoring of response-adaptive randomized clinical trials. *The Annals of Statistics*, 38(4):2218–2241, 2010.

G. A. Zielhuis, H. Straatman, A. E. Van 'T Hof-Grootenboer, H. J. J. Van Lier, G. H. Rach, and P. Van Den Broek. The choice of a balanced allocation method for a clinical trial in otitis media with effusion. *Statistics in Medicine*, 9:237–246, 1990.

Index

List of Designs

A

Adaptive Biased Coin Design (Adaptive BCD)
Adjustable Biased Coin Design (ABCD)

B

Biased Coin Design (BCD)
Biased-Coin Play-the-Winner (BC-PW)
Birth-and-Death urn design

C

Completely Randomized design (CR)
Covariate-Adaptive Biased Coin Design (C-ABCD)
Covariate-adjusted Doubly-adaptive Biased Coin (CD-BCD)
Covariate-Adjusted Response-Adaptive design (CARA)
Covariate-adjusted Sequential Maximum Likelihood designs

D

D_A-optimum Biased Coin design (D_A-BCD)
Doubly-adaptive Biased Coin Design (D-BCD)
Doubly-Adaptive Weighted Difference design (DAWD)
Drop-the-Loser (DL)

E

Efficient Randomized Adaptive DEsign (ERADE)
Ehrenfest urn Design (ED)

F

Failure Driven Design (FDD)

G

Generalized Biased Coin Design (GBCD)
Generalized Drop-the-Loser (GDL)
Generalized Friedman's Urn (GFU)
Generalized Polya Urn (GPU)
Geometric Up-and-Down (Geometric U&D)
Group Up-and-Down (Group U&D)

K

k-in-a-row design (KR)